The National
Childbirth
Trust

NCT

Help Your Baby to Sleep

The National
Childbirth
Trust
NCT

Help Your Baby to Sleep

Penney Hames

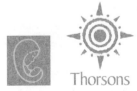

Thorsons

An Imprint of HarperCollins*Publishers*

in collaboration with National Childbirth Trust Publishing

For Richard, Beany and Richard (Junior), with love

Thorsons/National Childbirth Trust Publishing
Thorsons is an imprint of HarperCollins*Publishers*
77–85 Fulham Palace Road,
Hammersmith, London W6 8JB

The Thorsons website address is:
www.thorsons.com

and *Thorsons*
are trademarks of
HarperCollins*Publishers* Ltd

First published in collaboration
with National Childbirth Trust Publishing 1998
This revised edition published 2002

10 9 8 7 6 5 4 3 2 1

© NCT Publishing 1998, 2002

Original photography: Anne Green-Armytage, © 2002 NCT Publishing
Additional photography: Michael Bassett pages vi, viii

Penney Hames asserts the moral right to be
identified as the author of this work

A catalogue record of this book is
available from the British Library

ISBN 0 00 713605 6

Printed and bound in Great Britain by
Martins the Printers Ltd, Berwick upon Tweed

Contents

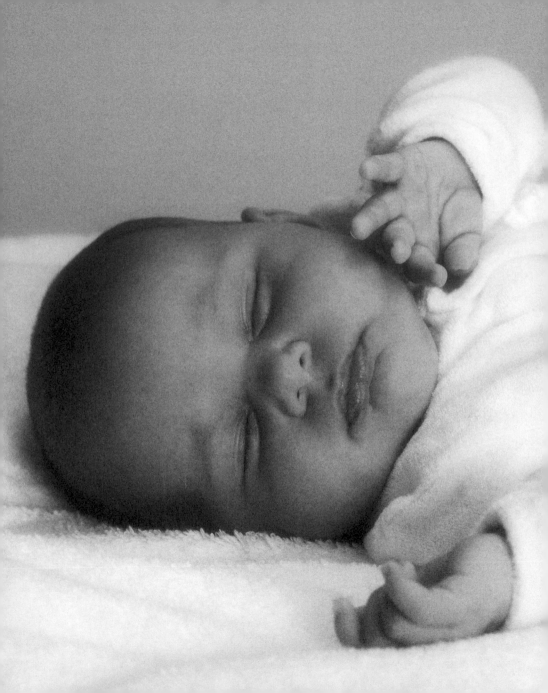

About the Author

Penney Hames, MA, trained first as a journalist and later as a clinical child psychologist. She deferred any practical application of either skill until after a lengthy research and development phase conducted on her own two children, Beany and Richard, and simultaneous years spent writing for the NCT's various national publications on the experiences of parents and babies. She is co-author of the NCT *Complete Book of Baby Care* and author of *Toddler Tantrums*. Penney Hames has represented the NCT on the All Party Parliamentary Group on Parenting, and now combines writing with child guidance work in Hampshire.

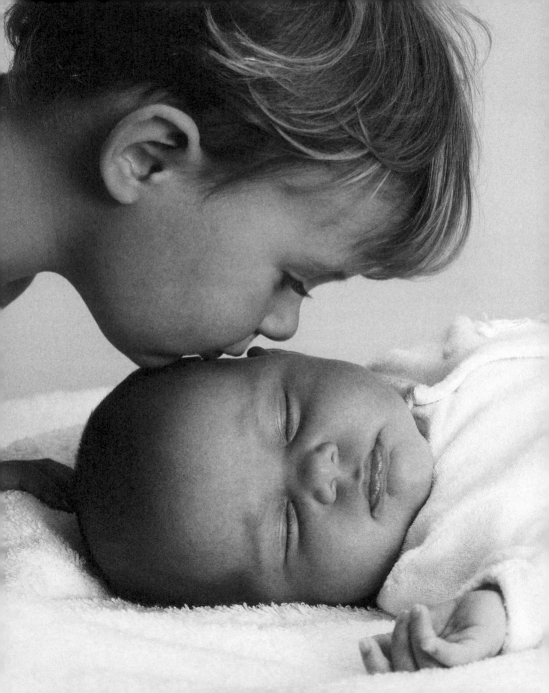

Acknowledgements

This book is the result of a great many hours on the telephone, and a great many more pondering over coffee and biscuits. Thank you to the numerous researchers and practitioners who generously and gently pointed out the subtleties hiding behind my first crude ramblings: Terry Cubitt, Dilys Daws, Patricia Donnithorne, Wendy Van Den Hende, Mary Kasper, Mary Nolan, Lyn Quine, Mary Smale, Pam Stretch, Martin Taylor, June Tranmer, Graham Tyler, Luci Wiggs, Olwen Wilson, Dieter Wolke, Anne Wynne-Simmons, Samantha Sherratt. Thanks also to my editor, Daphne Metland, for supplying the mountain which prompted my steep learning curve – I've loved every minute.

I'd also like to thank my own children, Beany and Richard, for giving me ample nocturnal opportunities to consider my own sleep strategies over the last nine years, and showing me that sleep confidence is contagious. If only I'd known at the time that all that night-time activity was research for a book I might have applied for a grant. Thanks also to my husband, Richard for fitting my tottering explanations into the broader scope of a theory of human development, and also for getting a job at the other end of the country so that I could use the computer during the week – you can come back now.

But most importantly of all I'd like to say thank you to all the parents quoted in this book, and the many other parents who talked to me, but whom I didn't have space to quote. Without your expert knowledge of what worked (and didn't work) in practice for your family, this book would have been impossible. Sleeping problems, our reactions to them, and the ways we deal with them are as diverse as the relationships that we build with our babies, and like those relationships need gentle and very personal consideration.

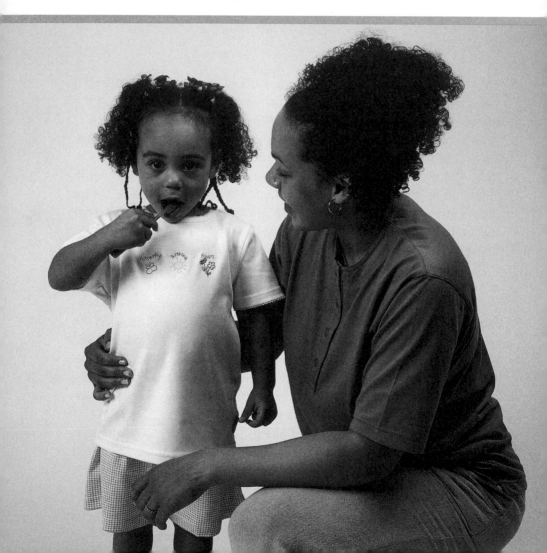

Introduction

Sleepless babies are all too common. One small paragraph in *New Generation*, the Journal of the National Childbirth Trust, which asked for parents' experiences for this book elicited dozens of replies. Then, talking to an astonishing array of professionals and researchers who have devised, through their widely differing disciplines, effective approaches or remedies for the sleeplessness of babies led me on to dozens more women. And women who had heard about the book on the grapevine of my local National Childbirth Trust branch, also called. Find me a parent and I'll show you someone with an opinion about babies' sleep.

The problem with any subject worth its salt is that right-minded, sensitive people can believe any number of threateningly different things. I believe that an author ought to listen to all these different opinions, try to see the value in each, and while rejecting none, chart a clear course for each reader, irrespective of how that reader prefers to travel.

So much for the theory. I'm sure that my own persuasions are written large in between the lines of this book. Nevertheless I hope that *Help Your Baby to Sleep* has accomplished three things: first, to acknowledge that no one approach is right for everybody; second, to accept that complex emotional ties may make the supposedly simple act of leaving your baby to sleep heart-wrenchingly difficult, and that is not simply something to overcome, but an awareness that may suggest a different approach; and third, to express the ambivalence and complexity of a vast range of attitudes, through the words of parents.

I hope you find in it something that speaks to you.

Penney Hames

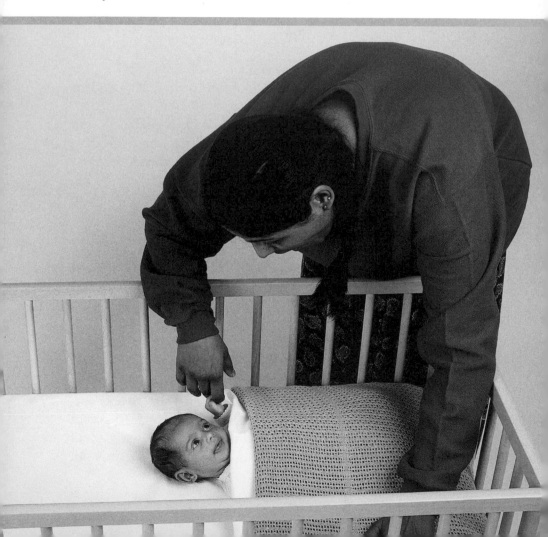

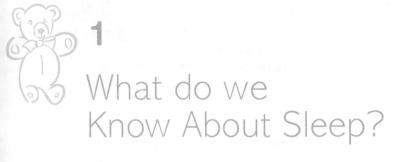

1

What do we Know About Sleep?

Oh sleep! It is a gentle thing, beloved from pole to pole

Coleridge, 'The Ancient Mariner'

Why does my Baby Sleep so Much?

Babies have a lot to learn, and quickly. But it's hard to reflect on anything when there's a lot going on. This is one of the reasons that babies sleep so much. Putting the world into some sort of order takes a bit of peace and quiet. While he is asleep your baby's brain can organize the vast array of experiences he has when he's awake. At the same time, chemicals in the brain and body are renewing themselves ready for more activity. As new parents we also have a lot to learn, and we also need our sleep to help us do it. Without sufficient sleep everyone suffers.

How Much Sleep does a Baby Need?

Most of us come to parenthood better prepared for the birth than for life with our baby. Charlie felt unsure and desperate for sleep when Elisa was tiny:

> *Elisa's two weeks and three days and she doesn't have a routine yet. Her best night was when she slept for three hours and then fed for one-and-a-half hours. I'd really like her to feed and then sleep for four hours.*

It can be a fraught time. You don't know what to expect, everyone else seems to have it sussed, and you are just so tired ... Sometimes it's helpful if you know about the average baby so that you stop expecting your baby to sleep for longer or more regularly than most babies manage. When Charlie found out that Elisa's little-and-often-never-at-the-same-time-twice approach to sleep was the standard new baby format, she began to relax.

Naturally, sleep researchers have discovered average sleep needs for babies of different ages (see below). But treat them with care. There are wide variations between one baby's need for sleep and another's. Just because your baby doesn't sleep as much as the average doesn't mean that there is something wrong. After all, any average figure means that half will be below and half above. And don't worry that your baby's erratic sleep is harming him. In his first few months a healthy baby will take as much sleep as he needs; he won't be able to help himself.

Some new-born babies sleep 21 out of 24 hours. Others, with less feeling for their parents, need as little as eight hours; the average at birth is about 16 (about two-thirds of the 24-hour day), and gradually falls to about 14 hours by one year.

Average Number of Hours of Sleep Needed

Age	Daytime	Night-time
1 week	8	8½
4 weeks	6¾	8¾
3 months	5	10
6 months	4	10
9 months	2¾	11¼
12 months	2½	11½
2 years	1¼	11¾
3 years	1	11
4 years	–	11½
5 years	–	11

(Quine 1997)

It doesn't matter whether your child is hitting these averages – some children sleep for longer and some for less. The acid test is whether your baby wakes happy and alert. If he does, you know he's had enough sleep; if he seems irritable or tired, he may need to sleep longer.

Our oldest son, Robert, has the sleep requirements of Mrs Thatcher. If you hand our youngest, Jonathan, a nappy at 6.30–7pm he will take himself to bed '

Cathy and Adam

Jessica only needs ten hours' sleep a day. I remember asking at her six-week check-up whether ten hours sleep a day was enough. If she has a two-hour nap she goes to bed with me for eight hours. If she goes to bed at 7pm she will wake up at 3am and be ready to start the day, so it is easier if she keeps the same hours as me.

Yvonne

A Sense of Rhythm

Most adults and older children have a diurnal pattern of sleeping and waking – we sleep at night and wake in the day. Your new-born baby has no such pattern. He is missing two things: the physiological maturity to be able to do it and your guidance. Once he has developed the first, he can make use of the second.

By the end of the first month most babies start to fit in with the adult pattern. But a thorough going awake-most-of-the-day-sleep-all-night rhythm doesn't usually appear until three or four months when your baby's physiology is mature enough.

Breathing in Sleep

Babies often pause in their breathing for anything up to a few seconds at a time while they sleep. This is quite normal and your baby will spontaneously begin to breathe again. Often your baby of less than four months will wake as his breathing pauses, and this kick-starts his breathing into action again. As he matures, your baby begins to breathe more regularly, without pausing, and at the same time he wakes less frequently.

Babies are very adaptable, and amazingly competent, but at birth they still need a lot of physical, close and loving support from their parents to help them adjust to an independent life. Researchers have found that touching, stroking and holding your baby has a marvellous effect on his ability to regulate his breathing and his temperature – and that this is as true at night as it is in the day. (See Chapter 4 for a fuller discussion of this point.)

When will He Sleep Through the Night?

Maybe not ever. But waking at night and waking you at night are different things. Your baby probably wakes more often than you think. Most people, children and adults alike, come to consciousness several times a night, but some are able to soothe themselves back to sleep while others lie awake tossing and turning, missing that certain something that will allow them to drift off again. Babies in this second group soon realize how to get hold of that certain something. They cry and in comes mum or dad. It's not waking up that's the problem, it's not being able to go back to sleep again.

In the beginning almost every baby wakes and cries about five times a night, and almost every parent expects that they will. But by the time they reach nine months the average baby wakes only once or twice a night (Anders, 1978), and he may no longer call out.

How Common are Sleep Problems?

Very common. Somewhere between a fifth and a third of all families say they have a sleeping problem during the pre-school years (Messer and Richards, 1993). Of course it's not always the same children waking all the time. For example, only 5% of children have a sleeping problem which lasts from their first to their second birthday.

 At 14 months Erica just suddenly got it and slept ... well, like a baby at last. I don't know what we did but I'm definitely going to do the same thing with the next one.

Karen

The fact is that some sleep problems last for months, some for years and some come and go but, roughly speaking, sleeping problems fade away as your child gets older.

> With your first baby you go in with the expectation that the baby will sleep for four hours at a time, and you believe that you can be your own person in that time. When your baby isn't that sleepy you think it's you, or that your baby is weird, or that there's something wrong. At toddler group last week we looked around and everyone looked tired and we said how many of you have been up all night? I think it was about 80% of the mothers who put their hands up. You could see the other mothers, the other 20%, looking round and thinking: "What's wrong with my baby, why does he sleep?
>
> **Teresa, mother of three, who tried 'everything' with her first**

Although many children with sleep problems improve without specific treatment, many improve a lot more quickly with a little help.

> Some babies just do it, and I kept thinking: "He'll just do it." People kept saying "He'll do it when ..." and I kept living for those milestones.
>
> **Karen, mother of David**

Deep and Light Sleep

REM Sleep

- body twitches
- eyes flicker
- smiles and frowns
- 50% of all sleep at birth
- 20% of all sleep for adults
- older children and adults may dream
- occurs mostly in the later part of the night for adults
- learning is organized and stored
- irregular heartbeat and breathing in tiny babies
- inability to regulate temperature in tiny babies
- adults woken from this sleep may be disorientated

NREM Sleep

- more peaceful sleep
- 50% of all sleep at birth
- 80% of all sleep for adults
- no dreaming
- slow and regular heartbeat and breathing
- harder to wake from
- occurs mostly in the early part of the night for adults
- the immune system is boosted
- physical growth occurs

If you watch your child sleeping, you may notice that there are times when, eyes closed, he seems to be watching some particularly frenetic cartoon. Beneath his eyelids his eyes may flick from side to side and he may frown or smile and wiggle his fingers and toes. If your baby could watch you he'd see the same thing happening from time to time, though not so often. This is REM sleep, which stands for Rapid Eye Movement. This sleep state is also called active sleep. Adults and older children dream during REM sleep but it's difficult getting a straight answer out of a baby, so there is no way of knowing whether babies do or not.

New-born babies spend about half their sleep time in REM sleep, and babies born before 30 weeks' gestation initially spend a massive 90% of their sleep time in REM sleep; whereas for you and I, REM sleep only accounts for 20% of our sleep. The point about this is that most of the arousals your baby makes from sleep are from REM sleep. Which explains why premature babies wake more often than term babies and all babies wake more often than adults. However, don't lose heart if your baby was born prematurely because premature babies are often better than term babies at soothing themselves back to sleep.

As they get older, babies have less REM sleep and therefore wake less often.

When he's not in REM sleep your baby will, perhaps obviously, be in non-REM sleep or NREM sleep. This sleep state is also called deep sleep or quiet sleep. NREM sleep can be divided into four stages. Stages 1 and 2 are lighter, and stages 3 and 4 deeper and harder to wake from. You are more likely to wake up during stage 2 sleep than in any other part of NREM sleep. In NREM sleep things are more peaceful – no eye movements, with slower, more regular heartbeat and breathing. There is a theory that NREM sleep is the time when bodily processes are restored, when the immune system gets boosted and physical growth can occur.

- Just as active (REM) sleep is followed by quiet (NREM) sleep, so we have active and drowsy periods during the day as well.
- Look out for signs that your baby is tired and put him down to sleep then – it will be easier for him to fall asleep at this time.
- Start to get him ready for sleep when he is still in an active phase so that he can enjoy his bath and be dried and dressed just in time to feel drowsy.
- If you miss one drowsy period you may have to wait an hour or so for another, as the whole cycle takes about this long to complete.

Cycling Through Sleep

NREM and REM sleep alternate through the night in both adults and babies. Babies cycle between the different types of sleep faster than adults. At birth it takes your baby about 50–60 minutes to complete a cycle, whereas it takes you about 90 100 minutes. The reason that this matters is that as you come out of REM sleep, ready to drop back down into NREM sleep, you arouse briefly. Your baby does the same. These brief arousals may or may not become complete awakenings depending on what you or your baby make of being awake alone.

Naturally, as your baby moves through the REM/NREM sleep cycle once every 50–60 minutes there's a chance that he could wake you every 50–60 minutes. What's more, these arousals happen with greater frequency towards dawn (Carskadon and Dement, 1989), just when you are having most of your REM sleep, the sort that helps you cope mentally with the day.

REM Sleep

- Pessimistic?
- Lacking in energy?
- Upset over trivialities?
- Can't see the wood for the trees?

Maybe you're not getting enough REM sleep. When you have a baby you may need more REM sleep than usual to help your brain 'organize' your thoughts and feelings, and file away yesterday's business.

People who are deprived of REM sleep for a long time become depressed and disorganized. They are unable to focus on what is important because they haven't been able to deal with the debris of the previous day before they start the next. Try to arrange things so that you can get a block of REM sleep at least every other night – you'll feel more energetic, optimistic and self-confident the next day. Try the following:

- Go to bed earlier than usual, so that you get to your REM sleep before your baby gets to you.
- Ask your partner to be responsible for the early morning shift from 4am onwards – at least once in a while.
- If you're breastfeeding ask your partner to listen out for the baby and to bring him to you in the early hours.

Researchers have found that when adults are woken while in light sleep it makes little or no difference to their day; when woken from deep sleep they tend to be a little tired; but when woken from dream sleep they find it extremely difficult to cope with their tasks the next day (Ferber, 1985, and Rotenberg, 1992).

Babies cope with frequent night-time wakings better than their parents because they set the pace.

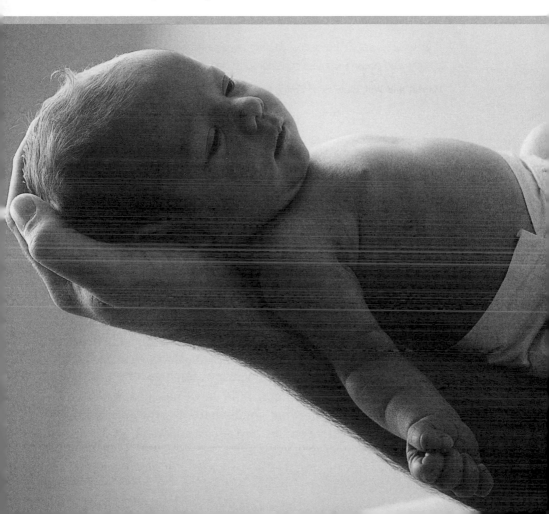

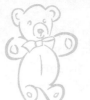

2

But What do You Want?

If you have a baby who sleeps, you are considered lucky, but if you have a baby who doesn't, you are considered to be doing something wrong.

Harriet and Will, parents of Emily, ten-and-a-half months

You can think that you've cracked it and that you know yourself and then you find that you haven't and you don't.

Buff, mother of four, who has an 'appalling' sleeper after two 'good' ones

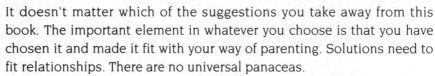

It doesn't matter which of the suggestions you take away from this book. The important element in whatever you choose is that you have chosen it and made it fit with your way of parenting. Solutions need to fit relationships. There are no universal panaceas.

What matters to your baby is that you have confidence in yourself and in him. But in the beginning, and especially with the first baby, many parents find it hard to decide how they want things to be, and what will work for their baby. Sometimes it can be hard just finding out who you are, now that you're a parent. Be patient with yourself – it will come. Confidence emerges when you know your baby and yourself well and are able to be loving and predictable. Most new parents find that when they relax and just do what comes naturally they become predictable. Loving, predictable and relaxed – it's a confident combination.

That Certain Something

Some people know how they want to handle their baby's sleep from the beginning. Melissa, mother of Jessie, read a book and was convinced:

> About three weeks before Jessie was born I read a book called *The Continuum Concept* which convinced me that the best way to sleep was together. It's been no problem at all since she was born. Sometimes Jessie's a bit restless and John has to lie on his front to protect his sensitive parts, but putting her in another room just seemed such hard work. After a couple of weeks she never really woke at night, she just goes around looking for milk. She sleeps through to eight or nine and sleeps really deeply. We have a 5ft 3in bed which is a great family bed. We built a big sleeping platform with rails at one side and the wall at the other. Possibly we are more relaxed because we don't have to think "Shall we let her cry?" I think our relationship (John's and mine) was improved because we both slept well.

Jane, mother of Thomas, Esther and Isaac knows what works for her:

> It was important for us to have an evening so we wanted the baby upstairs on his own, in his own space. Simon felt very stressed having the baby around him and I was very worried that I'd spoil the baby by not having a routine. I was happy for a little baby to lead me, but there came a time when I needed some time and I needed to instil some routine. So, from ten weeks once he had his bath in the evening, he didn't come downstairs. It was bath, feed, bed. It felt like we were back to normal.

Others know that they want to make a decision with their baby:

My itinerary is totally unaffected by Alistair's need to sleep. He sleeps anywhere and everywhere as soon as he's tired, and at night he sleeps with me in my bed. Even strongly disapproving grandparents have to admit that he is a charming, pleasant, well mannered and very independent little boy. Child-led parenting isn't a panacea, but it works well for a significant number of families. Too often "experts" seem to be trying to persuade us that our babies are tyrants needing strict regimes and hard-hearted discipline.

Monica

What all these families have in common is a sense of certainty. The parents believe in what they are doing, and in their baby's ability to fit in with it. It seems that babies who feel a sense of their parents' certainty sleep well.

Every time a new baby is born he brings with him an infinite range of possible relationships. For both of you it is a time of enormous change, and some of the changes may seem awkward and not 'you'. But by listening to your baby as well as to your inner voice, it is possible to smooth out most conflicts and to become confident of your ability to deal with any problems.

Listening to Your Baby

Take some time to get to know your baby and yourself. Do whatever feels right – gaze into your baby's eyes, massage his tiny body (more about this in Chapter 8), sing songs, tickle, talk about life, the washing up and the cat, but especially listen and respond to what your baby has to say. Once you and your baby know each other well he can feel how much you love him, and he will be quicker to respond to you. And you can relax, because you know that, whatever happens, he can cope and that you will be there to support him while he does.

I really don't think I was in tune with Laura as a baby. I don't remember knowing when she wanted feeding, when she wanted sleep. I think I relied on mum more for interpreting her cries. It got worse as I got more fatigued. I had a honeymoon period between three and five months, but then I got postnatal depression.

Sally, mother of Laura and Annie

Listening to Yourself

If you feel ambivalent about your baby's sleeping patterns it may be because you haven't acknowledged what your own needs are.

It would be funny if I wasn't so tired. The other day I was watching him through closed eyes so he couldn't see that I was awake. He was sitting in bed in between us and just playing and then he looked around and realized that we were both asleep, or so he thought, and he reached over and hit Mike on the back. Mike turned over and mumbled something to him and then fell back asleep. So, Jonathan turned towards me and whacked me until I "woke up". I thought "Who's running the show here?" I don't know. I'd like to have our bed back but Jonathan really seems to need to be with us.

Sarah, mother of Jonathan, aged seven months

Sometimes practical problems cloud the issue further:

> I tried to put her in her cot but she didn't sleep for long. I just didn't leave her for long. I couldn't get a routine because I had the other children, and sometimes I was doing different things. She ended up being in our bed and I think I wanted her there. I kept giving her targets. I said: "By the time I get to six weeks she'll be on her own." So I felt under pressure a lot of the time. I felt I was letting Pete down. He's not pushy at all, but every so often he jokes about it.

Kim, mother of Camlo, five, Evie, two, and Eden, nine months

And sometimes the way we live our lives stops us doing what we want even when we are sure what is for the best.

> When Bernard was seven weeks old my step-daughter came to live with us. As we only have two bedrooms and our lodger had the second, my step-daughter slept in the sitting-room. This meant I couldn't bring Bernard downstairs if he woke up. So, because my partner works long hours I would put him to me immediately so he didn't disturb my partner's rest. Now our lodger has moved out, my step-daughter is in the second bedroom and I can again use the sitting room at night.

Clare

You and Your Baby's Needs

Part of the job of becoming a family is to discover what you all need. Some parents meet their own needs vicariously by letting their baby's needs come first. This is how Pauline and Jeremy, parents of Hannah, Joshua and Martha, like things,

Martha has three or four stories and then one of us sits beside her bed until she is asleep, or outside her room, depending on her wishes.

And Caroline, mother of four, says:

I didn't have my children to ignore them. The health visitor just didn't understand that. She kept saying "What about you, what about you?" Well, I'm sorry, but my children come first.

Other mothers recognize that they need to meet their own needs first. Ruth, mother of Jess, four, and Alice, two, knew she needed her sleep:

I knew I had to work so they had to sleep. My going to work is not negotiable and I cannot function if I haven't slept. Both of my children have slept through the night from four to six weeks. From very early on I've put them down awake – from five, six, seven weeks. You could always rely on feeding them to sleep, but I decided I wasn't going to do that any more. I take them upstairs and I'm down in 15 seconds. A kiss and in the cot. I don't believe that any child needs to be fed and comforted every hour-and-a-half, and I'd be very unaccepting of a child like that. I believe there's a range of needs, but I don't believe that a baby has needs in the middle of the night. I think the lack of ambiguity is crucial – if they feel that they can stay awake then they will.

If you know you can't manage on five hours interrupted sleep a night, and want to do something about it, you shouldn't feel guilty. On the other hand, if your own needs are met by being available for your baby through the night then there is no reason that you should feel that those who choose a different method are doing a better job.

Certainly your baby needs to feel secure before he can sleep. But his security comes in part from your loving, relaxed predictability – not just from your presence. You don't have to be there when he goes to sleep and you don't have to leave him either.

What is essential is that you communicate your needs clearly, negotiate ground rules and stick to them. Don't try to be nice or to please. If you have to grin and bear it, something's wrong.

Discovering Boundaries

In the early days many mothers find that they love the enveloping closeness of their relationship with their baby.

When I fed Rachel and she sucked and slept a little and then sucked some more I didn't ever want it to end I just felt so complete – like we were still a part of each other and that Rob was some protective giant.

Kate

For others, unclear boundaries are more difficult.

The first months with Bryana were shattering and confusing. I'd waited so long to have her, but somehow it didn't feel right. I couldn't connect with what I felt I should be feeling as a mother. All the time I was sitting and "calmly" feeding in my mind I was frantically thinking how to be off doing something else.

Rose

After the first few weeks or months many mothers feel ready to put a little more space between themselves and their baby and many fathers are equally ready to develop an increasing sense of their place in the relationship. Many babies move from sleeping in their parents' room to sleeping alone at this time. Yet sometimes, and especially when you haven't found becoming a parent a smooth ride, it's hard to find comfortable new boundaries between you, your partner and your baby. Sometimes it can feel almost impossible either to put your baby in his cot and leave him to sleep or to have him in your bed without feeling guilty.

Saying goodnight to your baby can stir up ambivalent and powerful feelings, which may be difficult to face.

Sleep Problems May Occur When ...

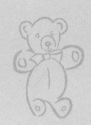

- You feel anxious
- You feel isolated
- You have postnatal depression
- You hadn't planned this baby
- You don't love this baby
- You feel as though you are abandoning your baby
- You haven't been able to grieve for a loss, maybe even a loss that is unconnected to the baby
- Your baby seems to need you to be there
- You have marital problems, or there is a lot of tension in your home
- Something from your childhood still bothers you
- You have been sexually abused
- You work outside the house during the day and feel that your baby is missing some important closeness which makes night-time separations harder to bear
- You feel that you ought to pick up your baby every time he cries, though sometimes you don't feel like it
- Every time you leave him he cries, and you can't bear to hear him cry

Most sleeping problems do not hide deeper problems, but where they do, a little bit of soul-searching and a lot of honest and open discussion may help. Talk to someone you trust. And be kind to yourself; ambiguity and confusion are often part of the journey to the most rewarding of relationships.

Some parents find that talking with a child psychotherapist helps. Child psychotherapists understand that relationships can affect sleep and that sleep disturbances can sometimes arise from unreconciled losses in the parents' lives. Sleep is a form of separation – a temporary loss – and can be a powerful reminder of other losses or separations which still affect us. Such reminders can hamper your ability to let your baby go. (If you would like to find out more about brief psychotherapeutic therapy for sleep problems see the resources section on page 149.) You neither need to hang on to your baby nor push him away. Sleep becomes an example of how you can love him and let him go.

Loving and Letting Go

If you would like your baby to go to sleep alone but find it hard to get out of his room, you may find that listening and talking to yourself and your baby in a certain way helps.

Why Should I Talk Out Loud to my Baby?

- Because sometimes you and your baby both need to hear how you're both feeling
- It helps you clarify what you want to say
- Things said out loud seem more real
- It can stop the same old thoughts going round and round in your head

On putting him down to sleep, try tuning in to how you are feeling and acknowledge that out loud. It'll sound funny the first time you do it but if you talk directly to your baby it may seem less crazy. If you want to laugh – go right ahead, it could be part of the medicine.

Describe How it Feels

To begin, think about how you feel as you are ready for him to sleep. You may feel confused, scared, angry, exhausted, or a hundred other emotions. Put a name to it. Tell your baby. Start your sentence with 'I feel ...' rather than 'I feel like ...'. So, 'I feel ... tired and scared' rather than 'I feel like ... I could sleep standing up and I feel like ... a failure.' Some people find that when they finally say how they are feeling, they start to cry. It's OK. Let it happen. Who's to know? If you start to cry, your baby may join in too. Give him a hug.

Once you've identified your own emotions it may become easier to listen to your baby's protest. Is it sad, angry, tired? Whatever it is acknowledge that that is how he feels and that you understand that this is a big, important feeling for him. You could say something like: 'You sound sad/cross/confused. It can be really hard to cope with big feelings like that.' You may feel strong and capable when you can hear your baby's sadness in this way. And he will be able to hear two important messages from the way that you say it: that it's OK for him to feel like this and that you will support him while he copes.

Explain the Deal

Next, try saying that it's time for sleep and that you have confidence in his ability to go it alone. True, you may not feel particularly confident that he can do it when you start, but just as you encourage him to feel he can do things during the day, so do the same here. In the day time you encourage him because you know he will do it in the end and you want him to feel good about himself. Going to sleep is also something he will do in the end and feel good about.

Finally, tell him when you're coming back. Be specific. He may not understand the difference between 'I'll be back in a bit' and 'I'll be back in two minutes' but you do and it will make you feel more in control when you say out loud exactly what you're going to do. Your baby will pick up a lot of clues from the way that you talk. But if you don't like the clock-watching approach, a good alternative is to say: 'I'll be here when you need me.' This is specific, because his 'needs' define when you come and go, and you've already shown that you are tuned into his 'needs' by listening to his cry. You are making a commitment to go on listening to him. Now start the behavioural routine you've chosen (see Chapter 11 for a range of options), coming and going as appropriate.

In this way you won't be abandoning him, but loving and letting go: a subtle but powerful difference, which will allow you and your baby to move on in your relationship. You will have really listened to yourself and your baby, acknowledged what you are both feeling and been clear about what has to happen now. It won't stop the crying immediately, but it may make you more able to deal with the tears. For more on listening to your baby cry, see Chapter 7.

What can I say to my Baby when he goes to Sleep?

- Tell him how you feel. For example: 'I feel tired/sad/angry.'
- Listen to his cry. Describe it to him. For example: 'You sound tired/sad/angry.'
- Let him know you care for him. For example: 'That sounds like it's a real problem for you.'
- Let him know what you want him to do. For example: 'I want you to sleep now.'
- Let him feel your confidence in him. For example: 'This is tough but I know you can do it.'
- Tell him when you're coming back. For example: 'I'll be back in one minute/in the morning/when you need me.'

Choose your own words if these do not feel right to you. Of course, talking to a baby like this may feel ridiculous. This technique isn't for everyone. You decide whether it's for you.

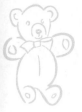

3

What does your Baby need for a Good Night's Sleep?

 Esme was born when our boy was five years old. Things had changed since he was born. We were much more relaxed as parents, and confident. We were also more aware of our responsibility and ability to encourage patterns of behaviour in our children.

Brenda and Dave, parents of Mark and Esme

It's a complex business. Your new born baby will need to be safe (see page 33 on safe sleeping), sleepy and comfortable – fed, clean and dry, warm and free of pain. But from about three months many babies are a little bit more astute and are ready to respond to a more definite timetable. There's a lot you can do to help your baby learn.

Babies like to understand, but they are not clever enough to grasp a lot of complications – they like things clear and they like repetition. So, to get your baby to understand the idea of going to sleep, you'll need to have a few clear steps and to go about it in the same way every time (see pages 28–32 for some tips about the end of the day, bedtime routines and sleep associations).

Organizing the Day

Strange as it may seem, having a regular breakfast time has a lot to do with getting a good night's sleep. Babies don't fit naturally into the daily pattern of sleeping and waking that we adults take for granted, so if you have a *laissez-faire* attitude to the day, with moveable feasts and naps when needed, your child might develop the same attitude to bedtimes and night wakings.

I really don't know why Sophie slept through the night from very early – luck maybe! However, I do feel a bedtime routine is essential and even some kind of routine during the day.

Diane, mother of Sophie, aged 15 months

Many parents find that thinking about the patterns they create during the day as well as at night helps their baby to develop a more regular routine. You may find that a structured day with meals and naps at fairly regular times, give or take ten minutes, gives your child a better chance of a regular bedtime with continuous sleep. If your baby is bathed, fed and sleepy by 6pm, it's best not to keep him awake waiting for daddy to come home for a cuddle, especially if that could be any time up to 9pm. This doesn't mean being ruled by the clock. Some days are bound not to fit your pattern. But knowing what your goal is, allows you to respond to your child's needs while recognizing that flexible routines can provide a reassuring anchor.

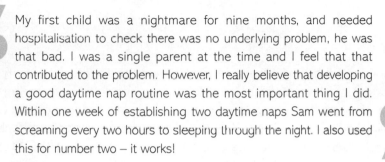

> My first child was a nightmare for nine months, and needed hospitalisation to check there was no underlying problem, he was that bad. I was a single parent at the time and I feel that that contributed to the problem. However, I really believe that developing a good daytime nap routine was the most important thing I did. Within one week of establishing two daytime naps Sam went from screaming every two hours to sleeping through the night. I also used this for number two – it works!

Fiona

However, some parents feel that routines can get in the way of meeting their own and their children's needs, and stop them responding to their child as an individual. Many of these parents prefer their children to eat and sleep wherever and whenever they like.

> By the time he was five months old Thomas occasionally slept through the night. But reading *The Continuum Concept* made me realize I did feel odd about the hours of separation from him. I decided to continue to sit up and feed him and gently put him in his cot in the evening. When he woke in the night I'd follow how I felt or how he seemed to feel and either take him in with me or to the guest-room double bed for a feed and sleep or just sit up to feed him to sleep again and pop him back in the cot. The sleeping through stopped immediately. But I feel it worked because I gave myself to him 101% instead of getting annoyed. When he'd perk up after an hour's feed from 8pm to 9pm and I'd felt he was just dropping off, I'd laugh and say, "Well we'd better go downstairs and see what daddy's doing." The key was to be really and truly willing to share his joy of life.

Sarah

Psychologists have discovered that when adults live in a laboratory for a few days without a watch or clock or any other way of discovering the time, they tend to sleep longer and stay awake longer so that they quickly become out of sync with the outside world. In fact, adults' biological clocks are set to run on a 25-hour clock and not the 24 into which we squeeze ourselves. This is why we find it easier to stay up late at night than to go to bed earlier than usual.

Your baby's internal clock is set to the same rhythm. If you let him he could gradually work his way round to an increasingly late bedtime and late morning wakening.

Bedtime Routines

If you want your baby to go to sleep at a regular time, the best way to complete a well-organized day is with a bedtime routine. When you look into your baby's eyes around the time of the six-week check-up there finally seems to be someone home – or almost. So this is a good time to introduce a bedtime routine if you haven't already done so. In fact, many babies begin to sleep a lot better from this point without much prompting and many have developed a definite pattern of their own making by the time they are three or four months old.

A bedtime routine will probably include some or all of the following: bath, feed, story or quiet play, cuddle and a kiss. And it will end with your baby in his place for sleep on his own or with you. A bedtime routine can be as long or as short as you like. Many people find saying goodbye difficult. A bedtime routine can be a good way of preparing you and your baby for the separation of sleep.

> It took me a couple of weeks to get myself organized and then we decided to organize Thomas. Lots of people had given us advice. So we decided to have a set bedtime to have the evening to ourselves. We started with a bath, and then into the bedroom with a very dim light so that we could just see, for his last feed. He slept through the night at six weeks.

Sue, mother of Thomas, aged two

The main points to consider when developing a routine are:

- Is it peaceful? Waiting for a partner to come home from work for half an hour of rough-and-tumble play can be counterproductive. Save it for the weekend.
- Do all the elements always come in the same order? Babies feel more relaxed when they can predict what's coming next.
- Is it practical? Sometimes a family will develop a routine that is useful at times and difficult at others – such as letting the baby fall asleep in front of the television or while driving round in the car. It is worth persevering with a more practical alternative if you can find one.
- Is it possible to do all these things within the time you've set? Starting a lengthy routine at 6.30pm for a bedtime of 7pm is doomed to failure. Experts now recommend a daily 20-minute dose of book sharing even with the youngest of babies, so it may be worth winding things down a little earlier than you had planned.
- Is anything else going to interfere with the routine? This should be a relaxing and close time for both of you. So, record that soap opera for later and ask your mum to call after your baby is asleep. You and your baby both need to give and receive full attention, so that you can both feel secure enough to say goodnight.
- Is there an end to the routine? Cycling through the last couple of elements again and again can be exhausting and frustrating for you

and suggests that your baby has not made the association between the end of the routine and sleep. Many parents find that whenever they put their child down to sleep he cries out, so they sing another song, or give another cuddle or drink only to find that the baby cries again when he is put down. A good routine ends with the baby falling asleep without you performing any encores.

Sally, mother of Emily, four, and Jack, 18 months, remembers that Jack used to be afraid when the lights were suddenly turned off. Now she ends their routine by getting Jack to 'blow' the light out himself with a little help from his bedtime friends, Piglet and Pooh.

Inevitably, there will be times when your routine has to go by the board – holidays, illness, visitors staying overnight. But the sooner you can reinstate the familiar routine, the more easily you will both rediscover your pattern of sleep. Alternatively, some parents find that where sleeping problems have already developed, a break in the usual routine can mean a chance to create a new pattern.

Kathy, mother of Lily, six, Robert, four, and Alice, two, delayed going away because Alice woke nightly and would only accept her:

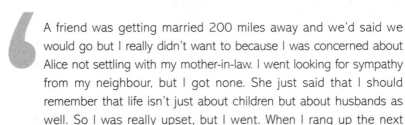
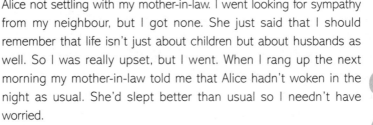

A friend was getting married 200 miles away and we'd said we would go but I really didn't want to because I was concerned about Alice not settling with my mother-in-law. I went looking for sympathy from my neighbour, but I got none. She just said that I should remember that life isn't just about children but about husbands as well. So I was really upset, but I went. When I rang up the next morning my mother-in-law told me that Alice hadn't woken in the night as usual. She'd slept better than usual so I needn't have worried.

Sleep Associations

As the name suggests, 'sleep associations' are the things your baby associates with going to sleep. The fact is that, whatever your baby is used to when he falls asleep in the evening, he may need again to get himself back to sleep if he wakes in the night.

Babies are incredibly adaptable – if you always sheared sheep in your baby's bedroom whenever you wanted him to sleep, he would still sleep – he would just learn to associate sleep with the sound of bleating and sheep clippers. And you'd have to be ready to fleece another from your flock each time he woke at night. Most parents find that a teddy and a goodnight kiss work just as well.

After the first few months of life, a baby who routinely falls asleep on his own in a room that is fairly dark and quiet will recognize the same conditions when he wakes for the average five times a night – and so be able to return himself to sleep without needing you. Some parents start a routine earlier than others:

James and Richard have both slept well from the beginning. I put it down to some advice I had at the start. The first night home with James I didn't get a bit of sleep, and then there was a knock at the door and it was the midwife. "Stick him on," she said "Hmm, he's just using you as a dummy. Put him down. Go and play some music that you like." We were a bit hesitant but did as we were told. It was the best advice I've ever had. He cried for ten minutes and then went to sleep. The midwife said, "When he's fed and you know he's satisfied, put him down." He slept through the night by the time he was six weeks old. It was the same with Richard.

Frances and Stuart

On the other hand, a baby who routinely falls asleep in your arms or at your breast will need to find a nipple and someone to hold him at night to do the same. Many parents who prefer this way of saying good-night to their baby are also happy to share their beds with them, so that they can easily recreate the evening's sleeping conditions:

> In the evening I undress Sophie, sometimes she has a shower or a bath and then we lie down in bed, read a story and then she holds my breast and falls asleep. I've had her in bed with me since birth. I did the same with Sam and Rosie when they were smaller too.

Clare, mother of Sam, eight, Rosie, five, and Sophie, two-and-a-half

But if you like your bed to yourself, it's counterproductive to lull your baby to sleep in the evening with a feed or a cuddle – because you'll probably spend a lot of the night in his bedroom doing the same thing again. If you want to spend your nights in your own bed with only adult company, sooner or later you'll have to get your baby to go into his cot awake and alone in the evening.

Sleep associations can take a while to learn. Especially in the early days, it may be difficult to identify a strategy that works. Sometimes, putting him in his cot and leaving him to it makes him nod off and at other times he can remain determinedly awake through all 25 verses of 'Oh my darling, Clementine'. Still, it is worth persisting with a structured bedtime formula that you like because eventually your baby will find the predictability of the formula reassuring and relaxing.

Safe Sleeping

The possibility of cot death worries many of us. But there are things that research has shown help to prevent it. Making sure we follow the recommended advice may help to put our minds at rest.

Many parents buy a baby monitor so that they can hear when their baby cries. These are a good idea, especially when your baby sleeps out of ear-shot. But there's another sort of device called a 'breathing monitor' which is designed to sound only when your baby stops breathing. The Foundation for the Study of Infant Deaths recommends that you only buy one of these breathing monitors if your baby has problems breathing. Talk to your doctor or health visitor before buying this type of monitor. In tests, parents found that breathing monitors tended to sound when there was no problem with the baby – making them more anxious rather than less. Parents also tend to check their baby less often when there is an alarm in the room, which means that they may not pick up the other predictor of cot death – that their baby is too hot.

Babies of less than four months old are less able to adapt to swings in temperature than the rest of us and need help to keep a steady temperature. Overheating can lead to cot death. So don't use any bedclothes that make it difficult to regulate your baby's body heat. Duvets and lambswool fleeces are out, but sheets and blankets are in. Babies regulate their temperature by losing heat from their heads so don't dress him in a hat to sleep. Your baby can also wriggle his head under a cot bumper, soft toy or pillow, so it's best not to put any of these into the cot until he is one year old.

We worried about having the duvet on our bed and that she would overheat but we'd move the pillow out of the bed and there would be an air space between us.

Sally, mother of Laura and Annie

Other co-sleeping parents regulate their babies' temperature by swopping their duvets for sheets and blankets and dressing their baby in fewer clothes.

The Foundation for the Study of Infant Deaths recommends:

- Laying your baby on his back to sleep (he is not more likely to choke).
- Don't allow anyone to smoke near your baby or in the house.
- Keep your baby's room at about 18°C/64°F.
- Cover him with a sheet and cellular blankets, rather than a duvet. (A folded blanket counts as two.)
- Don't assume that, because it's cold outside, your baby will be cold; judge it by feeling him.
- Check your baby by putting your hand inside his babygro and feeling his stomach. If he's warm, that's fine. Too cold and add another blanket, too hot and you need to remove one. (Don't worry if his hands and feet are cold – this is normal.)
- Lie your baby with his feet at the end of the cot so he can't wriggle down under the covers.
- If your baby seems unwell, seek medical advice early and quickly.
- Have your baby in a cot beside your own bed for the first six months.

If you are a smoker, have taken drugs or are drunk, you should not sleep with your baby in your bed because this increases the risk of cot death.

Cot death is rare, so don't let it spoil those special first few months with your baby.

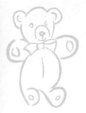

4

Where Should my Baby Sleep?

I think that children are supposed to sleep with their parents. Many of the sleep problems are to do with sleeping alone.

Margaret and Phil, parents of James, aged 20 months

Thomas went into his own bedroom pretty early on. I think he lasted about two days in our bedroom – we couldn't sleep. The health visitor had said something ridiculous like six months, but we couldn't keep to that.

Sue and Michael, parents of Thomas, two

For 95% of evolution, babies have slept with their mothers. Independent sleep is a relatively recent idea. So which is best – co-sleeping or independent sleep? As yet there's no clear answer but there is mounting evidence that our bodies are designed for close proximity or contact with our babies throughout the day and night until at least six months. It may be that solitary sleeping in the first few months of life makes too many demands on your baby's body, and that sleeping and waking within sight and sound of you helps him to adapt to life more smoothly.

Bed-sharing Benefits

The process works like this: it's not unusual for babies, and especially premature babies, to have breathing pauses, which last anything up to 20 seconds. It's quite normal. The breathing system is not fully mature at birth. If they happen in sleep, these breathing pauses lead the baby to wake and start to breathe again. Researchers have now discovered that babies who sleep close to mum and dad tune into their parents' breathing following a breathing pause and join in again at the same pace (McKenna *et al.*, 1994). There is also a suggestion that mothers who sleep with their babies tend to sleep up close, facing their baby most of the time and that this closeness stimulates their baby's breathing in another way – through the increased level of carbon dioxide they emit (Mosko *et al.*, 1997).

Something similar happens with body heat. New-born babies, and especially premature babies, cannot regulate their body temperature. So they can overheat. And overheating is one of the risk factors associated with cot death. Researchers have now discovered that babies and parents who sleep together work as a thermostatic unit. When the baby heats up, the mother cools down, bringing the baby's temperature down with hers (McKenna *et al.*, 1994).

Margaret finds another benefit: the rhythm of her waking and sleeping meshes with James's.

> James, who is 20 months, has always slept with us, and hardly ever fully wakes at night. When he was little he used to just snuffle around and latch on. If you are waking in the night, your sleep patterns coincide with your baby's, so you just gradually wake up with them. When they are in a cot you can't be so in touch, you don't hear them snuffling around. The first thing you hear is crying and that means you have to wake up quickly and they are already awake.

All this means that cuddling your new born baby at night is potentially valuable and not a bad habit, so long as you positively want to do it. After about six months your baby will be much better at controlling his own breathing and temperature, and will have cut down or possibly stopped his night feeds. So, this may be a good time to review how he sleeps.

Babies often provide clues about how they want to sleep. After a few months of co-sleeping, Ann noticed a change in William's sleeping position:

 He used to sleep right up under my armpit on the left-hand side, but by about eight months he was starting to sleep away from me and to move round the bed more, which disturbed me. I thought he might as well sleep in his own bed, so at ten months we moved him.

Anthropologists Wenda Trevathan and James McKenna recommend that you plug in your baby monitor the wrong way round, so that the sounds you make can be broadcast to your baby, rather than his sounds being relayed to you.

Their research shows that your sleeping baby can tune into your breathing, your movements and your talk and that this is good for his development.

If you are worried that you won't hear your baby when the monitors are switched, you could try a set of walkie-talkies so at least you can both hear each other.

But don't worry, this doesn't mean you have to share your bed with your baby. Even if you do choose a cot, your baby has ways of ensuring that you cuddle him at night. The average new-born baby probably sleeps in five or six different places during the night: his cot, his mother's arms as she feeds him on the sofa or the rocking chair, on his father's shoulder as he paces the floor-boards singing softly, and even the changing mat. In all these places he will receive beneficial contact.

Of course, most new parents buy a cot and then occasionally take their baby into their bed, and the advantages of a cot are fairly obvious. Other parents decide to sleep with their baby as a matter of routine. Others take the middle path of a cot with one side down butting against their bed, or a basket up close to them. You may want to consider the advantages and disadvantages of sharing your bed:

Advantages

- Less disruption to you, as you can meet your baby's needs immediately and easily
- Lots of physiologically useful contact for your baby
- Close physical contact can lead to close emotional contact
- Fathers spend more time with their baby – and many surprise themselves and love it

Disadvantages

- Baby wakes and feeds more frequently
- Less adult intimacy
- One of you is disturbed by the baby's small movements or his habit of lying across the bed, or on top of you
- Feeling that you never have a break

'Sex goes out the window when you have a baby in bed with you.

Sally, mother of Laura and Annie

'If we want to get intimate, John just moves her over to the other side.

Melissa, mother of Jessie

It is important to agree sleeping arrangements with your partner. If you choose to co-sleep, do so routinely, not just once every so often in desperation. If you do sleep with your baby, think about how you could give yourself more space. Ann and Simon kept their double bed and placed two chairs up against their bed while they waited for a Bed-Side-Cot to arrive. (A Bed-Side-Cot is a purpose-designed cot with one side completely removed which abuts your bed so that you and your baby can each have a space to sleep; you under your duvet and he under his sheets and blankets – yet within easy reach of each other. See page 152 for suppliers.) Alternatively you could push a single bed alongside your double one to enable everyone to sleep undisturbed – and to accommodate an extra sibling. Babies who co-sleep seldom choose to sleep in their own bed before they are two or three, and often much later, by which time you may well have another baby snuggling in too, although there is nothing to stop you moving them to their own cot or bed when you want.

If you are worried about the safety of co-sleeping use this checklist.

Is it Safe to Sleep with my Baby?

- You cannot smother your baby by rolling onto him in your sleep unless you have taken drugs or are drunk.
- The Foundation for the Study of Infant Deaths recommends that, until your baby is six months old, he sleeps in a cot next to your bed, close enough for you to hear him at night but without the risk of overheating under your duvet. They also recommend that you:
- Place your baby in the 'foot to feet' position with his feet to the foot of his cot so that he doesn't disappear under his blankets during the night.
- Use blankets and sheets for a baby under one, rather than a duvet, because it's easier to adapt them to the right temperature (18°C/64°F).
- Feed him in bed if that's comfortable for you but put your baby back into his cot once you are both ready for sleep.
- Do not co-sleep if you smoke, even if you do not smoke in bed. Smoking raises the risk of cot death.

Who Shares?

Of course, there are many variations on the theme. Some couples, like Clare and Chris, not only sleep with their children but stay awake as a family until everyone is tired, going to bed all at the same time. Other parents lie with their baby as he falls asleep in their bed and then get up and go downstairs again, returning later to sleep with him. Julie, who is single and the mother of Ross, aged three, did this.

> I felt I really wanted to give him as much time as I could at night and in the evening. I had to work all day, so we needed to be together at night.

Other parents co-sleep for part of the night, putting their baby to bed in his own cot and then lifting him into their bed when he cries. Some dads, and it usually is dads, end up sleeping alone just so that they can get enough sleep and their baby can co-sleep.

> Pete's been downstairs on the sofa bed with a sleeping bag for the last year. Occasionally he makes a joke of it and says he'd like to sleep with me again, and I'd like him to as well. He's very patient.

Kim, mother of Camlo, five, Evie, two, and Eden, nine months

What is Co-sleeping?

In some societies babies are not expected to sleep alone. This difference has a lot to do with how different cultures see the role of parenting. In Britain most parents see their job as helping their baby to become a separate individual. Most mums feel that at birth their baby is tied to them and that their role as a parent is to help their baby to develop, slowly and progressively, a sense of autonomy and separateness. Giving the baby his own bed and his own sleep space recognizes his individuality and will help to promote his independence. Every child needs to learn to be independent to survive in British society, so the theory goes, and therefore sleeping alone is in the child's best interests.

In other countries there is a very different set of assumptions based on what will help the child best adapt to the society into which he is born. The Japanese, for example, have a wonderfully evocative word for the utter dependency of the new-born baby. They call it *amae*. Amae means the baby's need to be protected and enveloped by his mother's unconditional love. Feeling the need to be protected and receiving this complete protection will have lasting effects on the baby. He will learn that we are all interdependent and that he has to harmonize with the group. A Japanese mother sees her new-born baby as separate, vulnerable and unprotected; her goal is to encourage her baby to become totally dependent on her. So Japanese babies sleep in company usually with their parents, sometimes with siblings or grandparents.

Most Japanese children sleep with their parents. About a quarter sleep on a mat beside the futon, the others lie between their parents. The Japanese have a word for the baby lying between his parents – *kawa*. *Kawa* is the Japanese character for a river flowing between two banks. The child is seen as 'flowing' between the two supportive parents. The imagery is powerful. What is a river bank without the river, and what becomes of the river without the banks?

Why do People Share?

Some parents interpret their baby's waking at night as a signal that he needs them. They take him to their bed as a way of meeting that need. Others feel that night waking simply means that their baby hasn't yet learnt to go to sleep alone and that if they just encourage him a little more, he will. Most of us occasionally abandon reason and will do anything if it just means we can sleep.

Some parents choose to share. Here's Julie, lone parent of Ross, again:

> Ross and I have developed a very warm and tactile relationship. I love him coming into my bed and snuggling in. My only worry is that I may make him more dependent on me, but I think it is countered by my lack of time with him generally, because I work full time. Ross does appear to be fairly secure.

Some parents want to share but have a baby who likes his own space:

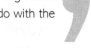

> We took our oldest son, Robert, into bed with us because he wanted to be held the whole time. (He was induced two weeks early and we've been told that induced babies like a lot of holding.) When number two was born we assumed that this was how babies went to sleep, so we took him to bed with us. Jonathan hated it. He went back to his swinging crib. Even now at two-and-a-half, when he comes in for a cuddle he wants just five minutes and then to go back to sleep in his own bed. It's nothing to do with us, it's to do with the child.

Cathy and Adam

Some parents want different things from each other:

> Eventually when Sam was 16 months old I put my foot down with daddy and took Sam into bed with us when he woke and was difficult to settle because I was a total wreck and couldn't cope any more with waking every hour.

Roslyn

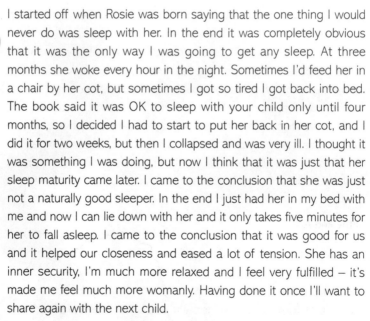

> My husband would be having them in bed with us, but I won't. He's softer. He was the one who was very soft with the first one, but then we were both tired and cross.

Liz and Adrian, parents of Hester, five, Bruce, four, Joseph, three and Isobel, 14 months

Some, like Catherine, begin to share as a matter of expediency, and end up loving it:

> I started off when Rosie was born saying that the one thing I would never do was sleep with her. In the end it was completely obvious that it was the only way I was going to get any sleep. At three months she woke every hour in the night. Sometimes I'd feed her in a chair by her cot, but sometimes I got so tired I got back into bed. The book said it was OK to sleep with your child only until four months, so I decided I had to start to put her back in her cot, and I did it for two weeks, but then I collapsed and was very ill. I thought it was something I was doing, but now I think that it was just that her sleep maturity came later. I came to the conclusion that she was just not a naturally good sleeper. In the end I just had her in my bed with me and now I can lie down with her and it only takes five minutes for her to fall asleep. I came to the conclusion that it was good for us and it helped our closeness and eased a lot of tension. She has an inner security, I'm much more relaxed and I feel very fulfilled – it's made me feel much more womanly. Having done it once I'll want to share again with the next child.

And still others have to share, and are relieved when they can stop. Brenda and Dave lived in a one-bedroom house when Mark was born:

> He didn't get his own room until he was three years old. He never had a cot, we didn't have the space. For a long time his night waking did not bother us greatly because tending to him did not involve us getting up ourselves. But after some time we did start to feel cramped and disturbed by Mark's presence in our bed or nearby. We were relieved when at the age of three we moved from our one-bedroom house to a three bedroom house.

Many babies who co-sleep like to lie on one or other parent's chest. It is likely that they are listening to the heartbeat, feeling the rise and fall of the chest as their parent breathes, and keeping warm all at the same time – something that will help them to regulate their own heartbeat, temperature and breathing in the first months.

Sleep Goals

Your sleep goal may be the same as others, but your journey to it may not. Ultimately most parents probably want their child to sleep in his own bed readily and with the minimum of help from them. For some parents it is important that the goal be achieved quickly, while others are happy that the process takes years and that the child will tell them when he is ready, and many more want to keep their baby with them at night early on and move him away when they all seem ready. Keep your goal in mind.

> Our ultimate aim is for India to sleep in her cot. But she is a brilliant sleeper, and I have no qualms about having her in my bed. She sleeps from 8.30pm to 8am. If she wakes then I'm there. I'm sure that she is happy to go into her cot awake because she is secure that we will go and get her if she cries.

Judy and David, parents of India, aged seven months

Sue wanted Charlotte to sleep independently from the beginning:

> Charlotte slept in a Moses basket in her own room at the start. The Moses basket was then placed in her cot from when she was about six weeks old. At 12 weeks of age she went into the cot and her sleep pattern didn't change.

Sam wanted Milly to be close for the first six months and to sleep in her own room after that:

> Milly sleeps from 8.30pm to 8.30am with two or three awakenings for her dummy each night. We consider ourselves fortunate. She was "sleeping through" like this from around ten weeks. I had her in bed with me for the first six weeks, then in a Bed-Side-Bed until six months. I think this helped establish a good routine and security for her.

Tips for Independent Sleep

- Put him down relaxed but awake.
- Make sure he is sleepy before you put him down, as he may be worried lying awake on his own. Delay his sleep if need be, and gradually bring his sleep time forward a few minutes each night, to fit in with your schedule.
- Be confident that he is able to manage on his own; it will rub off on him.
- New parents who are shown how to settle their babies to sleep alone and who believe that this is the best thing to do are more likely to have children who go to sleep alone and stay asleep all night.

Tips for Co-sleeping

- Discuss it with your partner first.
- Only do it if you want to, not as a last resort.
- Don't feel guilty if it's what you want to do.
- Do it every night and be prepared to do it for several years.
- Lay down with him when you have plenty of time to remain with him. You may find that when you remain with your baby while he goes to sleep, he initially takes a long time to settle because he is stimulated by your presence.

5

Feeding and Sleeping

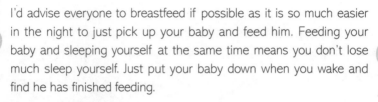

'I'd advise everyone to breastfeed if possible as it is so much easier in the night to just pick up your baby and feed him. Feeding your baby and sleeping yourself at the same time means you don't lose much sleep yourself. Just put your baby down when you wake and find he has finished feeding.'

Dawn, mother of six

'Our little girl, Gwenver, who is five, didn't sleep through until 16 months ago, she used to feed constantly, evenings, nights and all day. She was waking every half an hour. I did think about using a dummy because she was using me as a dummy.'

Sian, mother of Gwenver and Rowena

'With the twins my husband and I can never take turns. Mia wakes and cries so hard that she wakes Sam up, and so my husband has to get up. He finds it hard. Most of the books seem to encourage you to feed them together. I had an aversion to that. I just felt like a cow. I liked the idea of having a little bit of time with each of them. But this meant that I was constantly feeding one or other every hour or two.'

Kim, mother of twins, Mia and Sam

For about the first six weeks your baby drifts in and out of sleep and on and off the breast or teat. Newborn babies have stomachs the size of a walnut so at this age it is easy and comforting to feed your baby whenever he cries, whatever the time. Many babies, early on, do not even finish a feed in the way we expect but feed in clusters of small meals with big spaces in between, dropping asleep like the dormouse in the tea-pot, day and night.

Sleep Equations

In these first months when the nights are short and punctuated by frequent feeds, women who breastfeed definitely have an easier time of it than bottle-feeding mums. It's just one of the benefits. And parents who sleep with their tiny babies have easier nights than parents who have to get up to fetch a crying, hungry baby.

Breast + co-sleeping = maximum sleep.

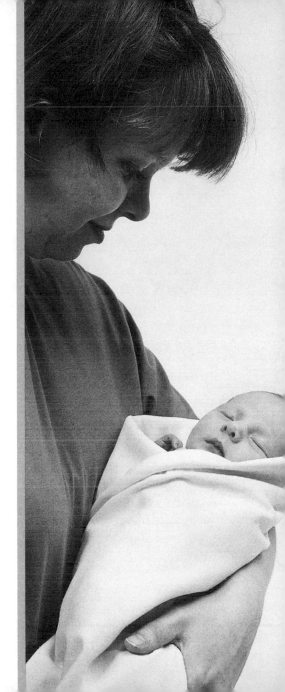

Breast or Bottle-feeders – which Parents get the Most Sleep?

Breastfeeding

- Partner can share by bringing you the baby/leaving you notes/bringing you tea/leaving a flask of soup.
- The milk is more readily available at night.
- You can sleep while you feed.

Bottle-feeding

- Lets your partner take a share.
- One of you needs to wake at night to make the feed.
- One of you must stay awake while your baby feeds.

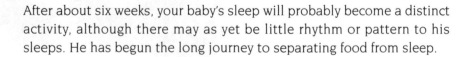

After about six weeks, your baby's sleep will probably become a distinct activity, although there may as yet be little rhythm or pattern to his sleeps. He has begun the long journey to separating food from sleep.

How about a Bottle in the Evening to Make Him Last?

Your breastfed baby may go through patches of needing to feed amazingly often in the course of the evening, cramming in as much milk as possible. He may be trying to get through the night, so go with it. Many parents try to short-circuit this extended re-fuelling by giving their baby a bottle of formula before bed, to help him to last. And this can work. Formula feeds are often heavier and less easily digested than breast milk, so your baby may stay asleep longer without feeling hungry. But a bottle in the evening may create more problems than it solves:

- If your baby doesn't suck in the evening, you will make less milk for the next feed.
- Sometimes a big 'bottled meal' last thing at night causes discomfort.

Some parents wake and feed their baby before they turn in for the night to give themselves a bit of extra sleep. It can work, but not always. Some babies may just take this as an extra feed, and wake up later anyway, while others refuse to feed on your demand.

 Someone said to me: "Put him on a bottle, he'll sleep better." But the little devil wouldn't take the bottle – he'd spit a bottle half-way across the room.

Teresa, mother of James, nine, Emma, six, and Mark, four

Alternative Sleep Cues

Your tiny baby learns that having a feed is the cue for falling asleep. Later on, you may want him to learn to fall asleep without a feed. The trick is to help him learn some alternative sleep cues. You could try tucking him in with a special toy, singing a lullaby, turning on his musical toy, sitting by his cot or popping in and out – whatever you both feel comfortable with, and will be happy to do for the next few months.

A week or two before you want your baby to sleep without a feed, feed him in the usual way and then if he has already fallen asleep, rouse him gently and go through the sleep cues you want him to learn. Keep it simple and do the same thing every time. After a week, you can cut out the feed and your baby will still know it's time for sleep, although he may take a few days to settle into the new routine. From then on try to avoid feeding your baby when he is tired, and use your alternative cues instead to get him to sleep.

Now Bernard is eight months old I am trying to get him to sleep through. I am doing this by not putting him to the breast when he wakes up – he is now offered water, and I walk him round until he goes off to sleep. The first three nights were hard. I was going to bed, getting up again a couple of hours later and not going to sleep again until 5am! But the last two nights he has not woken until 3am, and then only for an hour or so.

Claire

Try it in the daytime first – it will be a lot less fraught. Once you've cracked it in the daytime, you can do the same at night with confidence.

Having a tired baby fall asleep on you after a satisfying feed is one of the joys of early parenthood, especially when you can afford the time to just sit and soak up that contentment and peace. You don't have to give up this pleasure altogether. But, if you want to encourage your baby to feel OK about going to sleep without a teat or breast in his mouth, it's worth just rousing him a little as you finally put him down so that he feels himself drifting off to sleep without something in his mouth.

When Should I Stop Feeding at Night?

There's no right time. Some babies give up feeding at night, of their own accord, after a few weeks or months. Research suggests that the average breastfed baby sleeps through the night a few weeks later than the average bottle-fed baby, 13.28 weeks rather than 10.62 weeks (Wright *et al.*, 1983) while others go on feeding at night for longer – sometimes much longer. So long as you enjoy the closeness of the night-time feeds, there's no reason to stop.

 I still breastfeed James in the night and I think that that's helpful. I think that babies need food at night. He just snuffles around and latches on, while I'm asleep. If you breastfeed you release hormones that help you to go back to sleep more easily if you do wake up.

Margaret, mother of James, 20 months

But once you're no longer exclusively breastfeeding your baby it is possible to stop feeding at night and still meet his needs. Feeding on demand doesn't mean feeding every time your baby cries. It means feeding your baby when he needs feeding. The trick is to discover when he needs a feed and when he doesn't. It's something that comes with experience and knowing your baby. Kim found that Camlo, her first baby, seemed to need constant feeding – he would sleep for only 20 minutes at a time. When her second child, Evie, was born, Kim was better at tuning into what her baby really needed.

> I wanted to avoid lots of small feeds and subsequent colic (which in retrospect I think happened with Camlo). Evie developed a pattern of sleeping for two or two-and-a-half hours after a feed, then she would cry. After three weeks I tried to stretch the feeds out. I started to pick her up and just hold her. Rock and comfort her without feeding, sometimes for half an hour. Then she would go off to sleep again for another hour. Then I'd feed her. She'd feed well. Then the pattern would repeat itself. Later on I knew I could let her cry for a little while and she would eventually go back off to sleep. She soon went four hours between feeds – I couldn't believe this was happening.

Many babies wake at night, but can't get back to sleep, in spite of a feed. You may find that when you tackle the going-back-to-sleep part of the problem, your baby no longer wakes for a feed.

Mary and Peter found that their four-month-old daughter, Megan, slept better and fed less once they started a new routine at night:

'Megan has been entirely breastfed. I used to be up four times a night with her, feeding her back to sleep, every two hours, but by the time she was four months I thought she could sleep better than this. We tried the controlled crying technique where you leave your baby to cry for five minutes before you go in and reassure her and then leave it ten minutes before you go in again and so on, increasing the time between each short visit by five minutes. I thought it was a bit unkind and traumatic to do everything all in one go so I still breastfed her to sleep at night and then each time she woke I would go and breastfeed her again.

I got my husband to do the first two or three nights of going in and out because I couldn't do it. The first night was hideous – she woke and screamed between 2 and 4am. The second night was hideous as well and I was in tears. The third night it was better. And now she sleeps right through from 7.30pm to 7am and wakes up much more relaxed and happy. Having done it, I don't think it's cruel, but I don't think you've got to be nearly as rigid as some of the books say about sleeping and feeding on the dot, or you'd have a baby you couldn't take out.'

It's important to agree on your course of action first and to keep on reviewing it in the cold light of day. If you are a lone mother, why not try a new approach when you have a friend or your mother to stay? Knowing that someone else is there can help you to keep in touch with what feels right.

Sucking

Babies have a strong need to suck and derive a lot of satisfaction from it, and the more your baby sucks, the more milk you make.

But some mothers feel angry or exhausted by extended sucking, especially at night. If you feel this way, remember that it doesn't have to be you or a bottle that your baby sucks. It could be a dummy.

Alternatively, try shortening the feeds. The process is easier if you help your baby learn to fall asleep without a full tummy first (see above). After that, watch the clock for a few nights and see how long your baby really feeds and then the next week shorten each feed by about five minutes. Use your alternative sleep cues to get him back to sleep. Don't offer him more. Once your baby goes back to sleep easily you can make the feeds shorter again – it's up to you how much of a jump to make each time. Once you are feeding for no more than one or two minutes, you could try stopping altogether if you like.

Bottle-feeding parents can either make up less formula every few nights or make the formula weaker, by adding more water. By the time there's only water on offer, your baby may decide it's not worth waking. If he still wakes, don't offer the water, and after a few nights he may sleep through.

Dummy Facts

- Check that the need to suck on a dummy at night isn't masking a pain.
- Dummies introduced at birth may affect your baby's chances of successful breastfeeding, as they may change the way he takes the breast into his mouth.
- Delay using a dummy until after the first six weeks, when your baby's feeding is 'secure'.

If your baby sucks excessively night and day, he may be in pain. Most babies probably suck to relieve minor discomfort at some point (rhythmic sucking releases endorphins that ease pain) but a few need to suck for hours on end, night and day. Like Rosie, who sucked constantly and cried when laid down flat:

> Rosie wouldn't settle until one or two in the morning, and would wake up three or four times a night. I breastfed her until she was 11 months old, and it used to take me about an hour each time she woke. And then she had to sleep propped up in our arms because she didn't like being horizontal. Even when she went on to the bottle at 11 months she had to have a bottle each time she woke in the night. Eventually we took her to a cranial osteopath and he said that a couple of the bones in her skull were seriously misaligned, and she would have had a lot of pressure in her skull. She was sucking constantly and trying to remain upright to ease the pain. He treated her and within four weeks she dropped the bottle at night.

Dorothy

For more information on cranial osteopathy, see page 108.

Making Decisions, Feeling Supported

Feeding at night can be an emotional issue. Some men are happy that their partners feed at night because it means they can sleep; others positively support their partner's feeding, making sure that she has all she needs to do it well and even sometimes fetching the baby, and if necessary the bottle too.

Alistair left notes for Carol to find when she woke and fed Lydia at night:

> I'd get up to fetch Lydia from her Moses basket and there'd be a note on the rug saying something really slushy like "good morning to the most beautiful woman and the sweetest baby in the world". I suppose it allowed him to sleep with a clear conscience, but it was lovely.

But other men feel resentful of their baby – isolated by the intimacy that a mother and baby share while feeding, and breastfeeding in particular.

> We've had Rebecca in the room next to ours since the third day after I got back from the hospital. My husband just couldn't sleep. He said he didn't want her in our room when we were in bed because that should be our time together. And he didn't want me to breastfeed because he just thought it wasn't right and he wanted me back. So now she's in her own cot, with the door closed. When she wakes and cries for a feed I go and make a bottle and then feed her in her room, and put her back in her cot. I don't know, I suppose I'd like her to be a bit closer, but I have to respect his wishes – he is part of the family too.

Alex, mother of Rebecca, five months

Reshaping your relationships to include your baby can take great sensitivity and patience from both of you. See Chapter 9 for more on this.

6

Who Wakes at Night?

Everyone surfaces from sleep at night, but some babies and toddlers can turn over and go to sleep again on their own, others at some time or other and for a few months or more wake their parents for some help in returning to sleep.

Almost all children who wake at night are physically healthy, and are waking for a variety of developmental or social reasons; just a few wake because they are in pain or as a result of a disability. Whatever the reason, the solution to the sleep problem remains the same: decide what you and your baby need and how you want to deal with it and then get the practical help or support you need to carry it through.

There are many reasons for sleeping problems and each sleeping problem may be the result of many factors. Some parents are good at setting up a smooth routine that allows their baby to sleep. Others, and especially those who feel the stress of difficult relationships, post-natal depression, poor housing or money problems, find it much harder. If your baby is premature, ill, had a difficult birth, is a twin, has a disability, or cries a lot, your very natural inclination to protect him from any more knocks can easily lead to habits that may perpetuate his dependency on you for sleep. More than one of these factors and the chance of a sleeping problem grows.

You may not have started the cycle but your solution may continue it. Once established, sleep problems and tense, anxious relationships feed off one another. And it's a cycle that can spiral through the generations.

This explains why parents who had sleep problems as children sometimes have children with sleep problems. The link is stronger between mothers and babies than between fathers and babies. Both of Fiona's children woke at night and wouldn't settle without company in the evening:

> My mother told me that I woke every night until I was six and got in with her. I can remember being put to bed and getting out to play as soon as my mum went downstairs, and then having to scamper back to bed when she came up again. I didn't sleep well, how can I expect them to?

But there are things that you can try if you want. And you never know, you may just be helping your grandchildren to sleep better too!

Which Babies Tend to Wake their Parents more at Night?

- New-born babies
- Premature and immature babies
- Babies who had difficult births or are ill
- Babies with a disability
- Babies who cry a lot in the early months
- Hyperactive and allergic babies
- Twins
- Babies experiencing separation anxiety

Which Parents Tend to be Woken?

- Parents who slept poorly as children
- Parents with money problems
- Parents with depression
- Stressed parents
- Parents who go anxiously to their baby when he cries
- Parents who go to their baby as soon as he cries
- Parents who think they have a difficult baby

Some babies just seem ready and able to sleep through the night from a few weeks after birth; most babies take a little longer. Some babies learn to sleep peacefully and never look back, while for others each new developmental stage acts as a trigger for another bout of sleep disruption.

Help your Baby Sleep

How your baby's development affects his ability to settle himself to sleep.

Age	Possible reasons	What can I do?
0–4/6 months	Your baby may wake because of internal changes: breathing pauses, hunger, light sleep.	*Either* sleep close to him so that neither of you are too disturbed and he can get what he needs from you easily *Or* accept that you will be up several times a night.
7–8 months and 16–18 months	He may find separations hard to bear. He may want to be close to you day and night.	*Either* sleep close to him so that he doesn't have to cope with the separation at night *Or* show him that he can cope with separation at night (see Chapter 11, the kissing game and gradual withdrawal). Make a decision.
9–15 months and over 18 months	He may delay bedtime and wake you from habit. Maybe he doesn't know how to go to sleep on his own.	*Either* sleep close to him so that you can minimize the disturbance for both of you until he chooses to move *Or* show him gently but firmly how you want him to sleep (see Chapter 11, any behaviour management plan).

All ages are of course approximate. Your baby may experience these stages earlier or later than the average baby.

How Long Should I go on Accepting That my Baby Wakes me at Night?

It's up to you, but it's best for your baby if he can easily disturb you for the first six months of his life, and it may help him if you're available for the next six months as well. Babies need to wake at night in the early months for food and because their immature bodies need contact with nurturing adults at regular intervals just to keep going.

After the first six months your baby may no longer need to be with you at night for physical reasons, but he may still need you psychologically.

At about seven months your baby is beginning to grapple with the idea that you and he are not one and the same thing, as he originally assumed, but two different people. It can be a scary idea. Your baby's way of dealing with this is to stick with you more than normal. He may show more 'clingy' behaviour in the daytime and have difficulty falling asleep alone at night. And as he floats in and out of sleep at night he senses that you are no longer there and he may call out for you to restore the togetherness that he feels is the natural order. In fact, nearly half of all children who normally sleep through the night are disturbed in their sleep between seven and nine months.

Psychologists call this separation anxiety. It occurs at about seven or eight months and within a couple of months it passes. But it's not a once-and-for-all affair. Throughout his first two years your baby will have times when he will be getting to grips with his place in the world – and while he's doing that he'll need a lot of help from you. He'll need your reassurance, your encouragement and to feel your confidence in him. He may well want to be with you more than usual, night and day. How you deal with this is up to you.

This is why most sleep therapists recommend that you wait until your baby is a year before you try out any behaviour management plan which involves leaving your baby to cry. By this time, the theory goes, you can be sure that your baby is calling for you out of habit rather than need. However, there are behaviour management techniques that involve very few tears and can be tried even with a baby at the height of separation anxiety (see page 118).

Difficult Births or Illness

Babies who have had difficult or long births are sometimes poor sleepers too. Such babies often seem more irritable from the beginning, crying more and spending less time asleep than their contemporaries. They also go on to sleep less well than other children when they are older. Babies who have had difficult births may also have specific health problems caused by the pregnancy or birth which affect their ability to sleep well.

Janet's daughter Eleanor was delivered by forceps after a failed ventouse, and had a misshapen head and an eye that wouldn't close where the forceps had caught her:

I stroked the eyelid for a couple of days until it closed. But Eleanor never slept well. She moved all over the place, her blankets were all over. She found it hard to go to sleep and she was constantly waking at night and needing to suck. A year-and-a-half later, when her sister Anna was born, she saw the bottle, latched on to it and carried it round for the next year-and-a-half, sucking all the time. I can remember vividly one Christmas night at a quarter past three she had been screaming for two hours and her scream was going up a pitch at a time. I was at my wits' end. Finally I put her dummy in and within two minutes she fell asleep. A relative suggested cranial osteopathy when she was three. The osteopath said there was a lot to do. He said that all her bones were locked up, where they should move, particularly down one side where the forceps had caught her. She had tremendous pressure in her head, especially when she lay down. I explained it to myself by saying that the sucking would have relieved the pressure. The first day after the first treatment she wet the bed. It was a wonderful sign – it told me that she was asleep. Then one day, after three months, she just put the bottle down. It took us six months of treatment to get her to really sleep well. Now she sleeps 12 hours a night.

(See page 108 on alternative help for more about cranial osteopathy.)

Camlo was in an awkward position in the womb, at the mercy of strong contractions over a long period of time but without the right pressure on the cervix. I am sure the trauma he experienced in himself together with the high dose of adrenalin he got through my sheer terror contributed to his wakefulness later. Being prepared for labour to enable a relatively stress-free birth must be a factor in helping our new babies to sleep better. Also with a caesarean operation you are pumped full of drugs for at least two days – not a good sleep-inducing start.

Kim

A child who is ill or even just feeling under the weather may well have a disrupted sleep pattern. You're unlikely to succeed if you try to teach your baby new sleep habits when he is ill. It may be best just to go with it until he is better and more able to respond to your new routine.

Up until 12 weeks David had slept pretty well but then he went into hospital with bronchiolitis and they said we had to feed him every two hours day and night. So, of course, once we got home it was impossible to get him to sleep through. So we gave him time to build himself up and then we began the controlled crying approach.

Karen and Phil, parents of David

Children with a Disability

Many children who have a disability also have problems sleeping. But there's no simple reason. A few children with a disability fit into no recognizable sleep pattern. For example, severely brain-damaged children may not have sleep cycles and children who have less severe brain damage may shift quickly and unpredictably from one sleep state to another.

Children with Down's syndrome tend to have more sleep problems caused by breathing difficulties and to be more restless at night, kicking off the bedclothes and getting cold. And because a child with Down's syndrome is less able to regulate his body temperature effectively, this can be dangerous (see page 33 on safe sleeping and page 80 on practical tips.)

Often, however, babies with disabilities have problems sleeping because they are unable to pick up sleep cues or to relax enough to be able to sleep.

So for autistic children and children with severe learning difficulties who tend to have difficulty settling, to wake in the night and also to wake early, for deaf children who take twice as long to fall asleep as children who can hear and for blind children who sleep less well than their sighted peers, a plan that emphasizes sleep cues may be appropriate (see Chapter 11 for details about behaviour management plans).

If your child has any kind of diagnosed disability, you will probably already be in touch with the relevant support group. If not, Contact-a-Family – the organization that helps the parents of children with special needs – has an excellent resource on its website: The CaF Directory. This is an index of specific conditions and rare disorders that gives contact details of all existing support groups.

To share experiences and information with other parents who are facing the same difficulties as you are, really can help enormously. Get in touch with them via this Directory on the Contact-a-Family website at www.cafamily.org.uk

You can also ring the Contact-a-Family helpline on 0808 808 3555 from 10am to 4pm, Monday to Friday.

Some gifted children need a lot of mental stimulation before they are ready to sleep well, as Denise found:

Jessica is a very bright child. It wasn't until I made the connection between this and her difficulty falling asleep, staying asleep and waking early that I started to go out of my way to tire her mentally. To sleep well she has to be both physically and mentally tired.

Tearful Babies

Babies who cry excessively in the early months tend to have a problem with sleeping later (Bernal, 1972). This may be due to habit. The baby cries, the parents calm him by holding and rocking him – all quite natural and even sometimes helpful, but it establishes expectations for both the baby and the parents, and these expectations can be hard to break. Only you can decide when you and your baby are ready to move on.

Self-fulfilling Prophecies

Is your baby difficult? Does he cry at the slightest thing? Do you find him really hard work? Then take care. Psychologists have discovered that parents who think of their baby as difficult or unsettled, often become less tuned in to his needs and less willing to meet them. The result is that your 'difficult' baby ends up crying longer and harder than an 'easy-going' baby to get attention. He may grow into a demanding and difficult toddler. But there are things you can do:

- Try not to label your baby
- Concentrate on how he is feeling
- Give him the benefit of the doubt
- Focus on the good times too

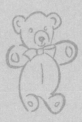

Twins or More

Twins can also present more sleep difficulties than single babies as Sue, single mother of Danielle and Sophie, remembers:

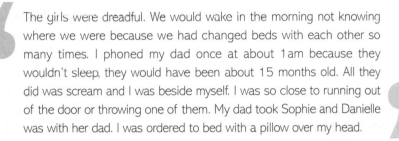

> The girls were dreadful. We would wake in the morning not knowing where we were because we had changed beds with each other so many times. I phoned my dad once at about 1am because they wouldn't sleep, they would have been about 15 months old. All they did was scream and I was beside myself. I was so close to running out of the door or throwing one of them. My dad took Sophie and Danielle was with her dad. I was ordered to bed with a pillow over my head.

Kim, mother of Mia and Sam, seven months old, feels that the anxiety of having both babies awake at night may have caused her twins sleep problems:

> When they were little I used to go in and feed whichever one had made the noise just to stop the other one waking up, but I think now that they were maybe just turning over and I should have left them. Or maybe if I'd had them in separate rooms they might have slept better, but everyone says "Oh! You can't separate them now! They've been together for nine months." So I put them in together and then went in at the first noise. We both still find it hard — the constant never being able to have a full night's sleep. And 5am is an early start.

Some parents remove one baby from his usual sleeping place for a few nights and try a new routine until they both start to sleep better, and others leave both where they are, try behaviour management techniques and find that the other twin sleeps soundly in spite of the extra crying for a few nights.

First-born Babies

Contrary to popular belief, first-born babies are no more likely to wake at night than subsequent babies. Any perceived difference may be just that – a perception. Many parents are more tolerant and at ease with the disruption that a baby brings second time around, and this colours their perception of his waking. One study found that fourth or subsequent children had fewer sleeping problems than other children, and suggested that this may be due to the mother's increased confidence in her abilities, or her lack of time to spend with her baby at night. However, not all parents have this experience as Ann, whose daughter Jennifer didn't sleep through the night in her own bed until she was six, explains:

Jennifer is our fourth child. The others all went through phases of sleeping in our bed/prolonged breastfeeding/night waking/late bedding, etc., but none like this one. All were sleeping through in their own beds by three years old at the latest. I felt jealous of parents whose children slept alone at night, resentful of her dominance, sad about our feelings for her being spoiled – and foolish.

Teething

Teething is blamed for a lot of sleep problems. If your child normally sleeps well and is suddenly disturbed at night it may be worth checking the gums and rubbing on a little gel. But if your baby wakes routinely for months on end, then the reason is unlikely to be teething. Try not to let teething disrupt your pattern.

> Thomas was starting to go about five hours in the night but then he started teething and we're back to square one – to every hour.

Ruth and Greg, parents of Thomas

> She isn't always a brilliant sleeper and whenever she has a disturbance in her sleep, it takes us about a week of being firm before she gets back into her pattern again.

Joy, mother of Sophie, who slept from six weeks

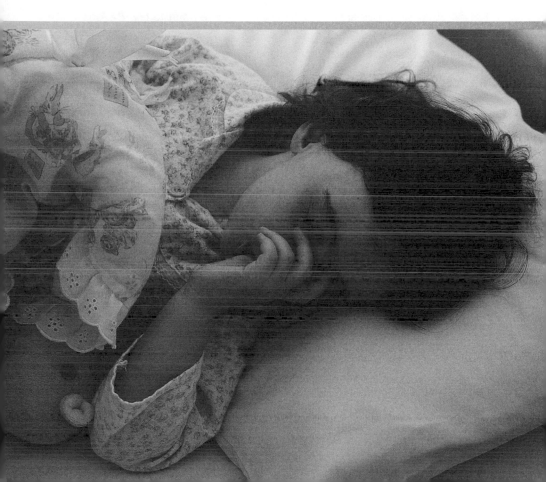

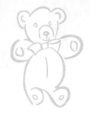

7

Crying and Sleeping

Ever since Bernard was born I have never left him to cry. The one
time I did I was in tears in five minutes. I figured that he would only
cry if something was wrong: hungry, dirty, windy or lonely – and I
was the only person who could make it right. As a result I have a
contented, happy baby who everyone thinks is wonderful. I am what
I would class as a very lucky mum.

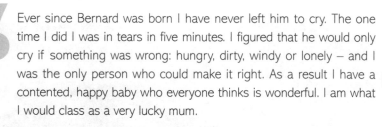

Claire

If it weren't for the fact that Adam cries so bitterly for hours on end
at night I would leave him to sleep on his own. But I can't ignore the
tears.

Sue

No parent wants their baby to cry, but all babies do, some more than
others. A baby who seems to cry endlessly, no matter what you do, can
be a shattering experience.

> This beautiful little nursery! She didn't spend more than three minutes in it. I picked her up, she cried, I put her down, she cried, I turned the washing machine on, she cried, I turned the washing machine off, she cried, I sang her a song, she cried, I bounced her up and down, she cried, her dad came in, she cried, her dad went out, she cried, the cat sneezed, she cried.

Victoria, mother of Helena, aged 20 months

Hearing your baby cry can be one of the most soul-destroying, anxiety-inducing, overpowering experiences there is. When he cries and there's nothing you can do about it, you can feel helpless.

But not everyone reacts the same way to their baby's tears. Some parents feel that crying is a natural part of the way their baby adapts to change, and leave him to calm himself, while others do everything to prevent their baby crying in the first place or to calm him when he does cry.

I can't Bear to Hear my Baby Cry

There are two different strategies that work well for different people:

Focus on the Crying

- Listen to your baby's cry – what is he really saying? Just keep on listening until you're sure you know, then relax and do something about it

Distract yourself

- Let someone else listen for you, and go somewhere out of earshot
- Listen to soothing music/relaxation tape on headphones
- Count backwards from a hundred before you go – he may be calming down by now

Two of the most common responses to feeling helpless are anxiety and anger, both of which can seriously affect the way you deal with your baby. Most of us have yelled at our baby at least once when he's woken for the umpteenth time that night, and many of us have lain awake just waiting for him to cry and then rushed in at the first snuffle. But most of us know that neither of these approaches work. It's knowing what else to do that is more difficult.

I'm absolutely convinced that nearly all of Helena's sleeping problem was me transmitting to her my own paranoia about leaving her.

Victoria

As soon as Camlo screamed I took him out. I didn't want him to feel trapped. I'm claustrophobic – I didn't ever want him to be in the dark.

Kim

Sometimes I'd just yell at her. I was up about five times every night, just walking up and down, or feeding, endlessly feeding. I was just shattered. I'd put her down and creep out and then she'd start again, and I couldn't take it. But it wasn't any good; she'd just cry harder and I'd have to go back.

Toni

Dealing with the feeling of helplessness can sometimes enable you to cope with the tears better, to reduce his crying and also to help him to sleep better.

If you have always gone to your baby as soon as he cried, being told to leave him to cry himself to sleep can seem cruel. But is it? Tiny babies cry because they need something: food, cuddles, warmth, stimulation – it would be cruel to ignore that plea. They also cry to protest at the unexpected, or at losing control – being put down, or as they fall asleep; opinion varies about whether it is cruel to ignore this cry. By the time your baby is seven months old a sleep problem may be aggravated by his fear that when you disappear you will never return. If you've never done it before, leaving him to sleep on his own at this time may be cruel, because it plays on his very real fears. Alternatively, see page 118 for a method that helps your baby cope with separation anxiety and yet sleep better.

Some parents, who suspect that they don't love their baby, feel cruel whenever their baby cries because they feel it proves that they haven't loved him enough, or that they have failed as parents. Such feelings make parents extremely anxious to avoid any crying, and can be difficult to escape. But remember, even babies who are loved cry. Loving parents show they care by accepting what their baby says and helping them to cope with the tears.

Doing Nothing is Doing Something

When nothing works, do just that. Some parents find that the less they do to help their baby dry his eyes, the more their baby likes it.

I put off trying a controlled crying technique for months, because it seemed so horrible. In the end we tried it and it did only take a couple of nights. I was feeding Harry maybe eight or nine times a night, a good night would be four or five times a night. I still carried on breastfeeding him but only last thing at night and first thing in the morning. That first night he screamed for four hours and then later he woke up, again for two hours. The next night it was the same. But within a week he was sleeping through. In retrospect I wish I'd done it a lot earlier.

Ann

It used to be thought that a mother or father who attended quickly to their crying baby rapidly found that they had a baby who cried less than parents who left their baby to cry.

The most recent evidence suggests that it's not quite this simple. It's not just what you do that matters; it's the way that you do it as well. If you are relaxed when you pick up your baby, even if you have left him to cry a little longer, your baby will eventually cry less than a baby who is attended to immediately by an anxious parent.

Probably the best advice is to go to him when he cries but take a deep breath first and relax, especially if you weren't quite ready for him to need you so soon, and then walk there. It'll be better for him and certainly better for you too. If you can't get to him immediately, don't worry, go when you can and relax on the way. He knows you'll come eventually.

The Surprised Cry

Most babies cry when they are surprised by a change to the regular programme. If he has been used to your continued presence as he falls asleep, your baby of more than a year will probably cry when you first leave him to sleep on his own. But if you do it firmly and gently, he will know that he will be all right. You are not trying to break his will; you are showing him that even when he is frustrated and shows it, nothing awful happens.

Maybe he will feel temporarily unhappy, but he will not feel abandoned or deserted, especially if you adapt one of the behavioural programmes in this book to your way of doing things. What is more, you may even find that he wakes in the morning more cheerfully than he has previously done. He certainly won't hold it against you. Have a look at pages 21–4 to see how to be kind to yourself and your baby while you leave him to sleep alone.

Many babies cry as they go to sleep, as you leave them or even while surfacing from sleep. But this cry may be a protest, not a plea. A protest at a change, rather than a plea to be picked up and stimulated again, and after a few minutes they settle to sleep.

What is he Trying to Say?

Most mothers rapidly learn to recognize their own baby's cry. But it may take you a little longer to sort out his different cries one from another, by which time you may have got used to reacting to his cry in a certain way.

When your little baby cries at night, you feed him and he falls asleep. Later, he cries at night, you feed him and he remains awake. It's time for a change. You need to begin to decipher his different cries and respond accordingly. If you can identify what his cry means, you will be better able to meet his needs.

Kim, mother of Rowan, three, and Lloyd, four months, has learnt that her baby has different sleep patterns to her daughter:

 At night when Lloyd cries out, I don't rush in at the first moan, it's just him coming to and calling in his sleep, I know that if I leave him he'll go back to sleep for 40 minutes or an hour, but when he cries again that means he really is hungry, and I go.

Positive Parents

Some parents don't like solving a sleeping problem by leaving their baby to cry even when he is no longer experiencing separation anxiety because they believe that the baby will feel helpless, rejected and frightened. Yet research suggests that, when following a behaviour modification programme to help their baby to sleep (like the ones in Chapter 11), parents rate their babies as:

- slightly more secure
- less tense or emotional
- more agreeable, and
- more likeable.

Maybe the babies hadn't changed. Maybe the parents just felt more positive after a good night's sleep. But this in itself is good news. A baby whose parents think he is agreeable is more likely to grow into an agreeable toddler.

Listen to the cry before you go. Decide what sort of cry it is. Is he frantic, angry, sad, hungry? Deal in the most appropriate way with that emotion. A hungry baby obviously wants food. But a sad or frantic baby may just want a cuddle. And an angry baby may just need to know that you are still around but that you expect him to sleep now.

Of course, a few babies cry at night because they are in pain. It isn't always easy to spot this cry, because it's so unexpected, but if your baby is in pain he won't be able to respond to a sleeping programme.

Something that helped us to cope when times were bad was changing our attitude, that is focusing on the fact that Ella was in pain from the colic and needed our help, rather than feeling that she was crying just because she was awkward! This made us feel sorry for her more than angry with her. Also accepting that we didn't have to make her stop crying (something we could only fail at) but just needed to be with her while she cried. In retrospect maybe this was a factor in Ella becoming more settled and peaceful.

Karen, mother of Ella, three-and-a-half months

Who's Crying Now?

Some researchers have suggested that some young babies may cry because they are attended to when they wake at night. It's an odd thought but the logic behind it goes like this. Every baby wakes at night and babies who have suffered difficult pregnancies or births or are premature may need to wake more frequently for a variety of reasons. Such babies are used to coping with a difficult situation alone, and don't know what to do when their parents want them to be a part of a caring relationship and so, the theory goes, they cry. If the theory is right, it may be worth leaving your baby who's had a difficult birth to cope with things on his own a little more.

Some psychotherapists believe that babies cry when they are unhappy or confused – when your baby has cried enough, he will stop and he won't be distressed any more. According to this theory, it's good for your baby to cry things through. So next time he seems inconsolable try just holding him and loving him without trying to make things better. Support him by staying with him and accepting his tears as calmly as you can. It may work for you.

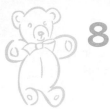

8

Practical Tips

If your baby doesn't fall asleep readily in the evening, wakes you during the night or wakes early, there are many things you can try which have worked for other parents, at least some of the time.

Toys

Toys are part and parcel of a happy environment for your baby. While he is still very young and unable to reach out and grab a toy for himself, it's best to stick to a mobile or musical toy strapped to the side of the cot out of reach, as large soft toys in the cot may cause him to overheat.

With older babies some parents feel that one or two toys are sufficient – cots are for sleep. Sue is sure that keeping it simple helps Charlotte, who has slept well from birth, to sleep:

The mobile, which plays Brahms's lullaby, has definitely had a positive effect. Charlotte has been used to this from the time the basket went into the cot. There are certain toys which she only sees in her cot, for example, a bunny, a squashy book and a spotted dog, and it is clear that she is delighted to see them and the activity centre (part of the mobile), when she goes into the cot.

Other parents feel that the more familiar faces their baby has around him, the better. If your baby is an early riser, a couple of special toys placed in the cot on your way to bed may help him to amuse himself for an extra five minutes in the morning.

A lot of babies become inordinately fond of one particular soft toy or object, and hold it tight at testing times such as when they are ill, or visiting new places, or falling asleep. Psychologists call this a transitional object – a cuddly which your baby associates with you and can bring comfort in your absence. Unfortunately transitional objects are often the least attractive of your baby's possessions. It's a humbling thought that a greying knitted rabbit with too much stuffing and only one eye is a substitute for you. Some parents introduce a cuddly from day one – at least this way you get to choose your baby's constant companion:

Thomas has a teddy that he won't go to sleep without. It always stays in his cot, although he does try to take it places when he has a cold. I just used to tuck it in with him. He sucks his thumb and holds onto the teddy with the same hand. If we go on long car journeys he has his teddy and goes to sleep.

Sue

Heat

We all sleep better when we are warm. These nights most babies sleep in babygros with the advantage that they don't get too cold when they kick off the covers or roll over. Baby sleeping bags are also available to stop your restless sleeper cooling down and waking up. To be safe, these need to fit fairly well, be sleeveless and have a low tog rating

(1.5 or less). A sleeping bag will keep your baby warm so be very careful about what you cover him with once he's zipped in – it may be enough on its own or with one blanket. Feel his stomach to judge his body temperature. (See pages 33–4 for more on overheating and safe sleeping.)

Aaron would completely strip off during the night and so become cold and wet. This then became his sleep pattern lasting a month. At this point I was so low I was even considering sedation to break the pattern. My friend recommended buying an all in one zip-up sleep suit put on back to front. BRILLIANT. The results were amazing and I felt ashamed that I had nearly carted him off to the doc's for sedation!

Gill

Noise

Some noise can be comforting to your child lying awake in the evening – it shows that you are still there. But sudden noise or sudden changes in the noise level may disturb sleep. You can reduce sudden noises from outside the house by installing double glazing or secondary glazing. A less radical and cheaper alternative would be to move your child to a different bedroom where there is less noise. Some parents have found that delaying the onset of the central heating in the morning allows them an extra half hour of sleep. If you or your partner rises early for work, take your shower or bath the night before.

Light

You can teach your child to be frightened of the dark, just as you can teach him to be relaxed by it. If you always turn the light on when you go to him and off when you leave he'll make the connection between light and company and dark and isolation. Try not to turn on any lights when you visit him, but if you have to – keep it low.

Many children prefer to sleep with a low light on, either all night or just as they go to sleep. There's nothing wrong with this. Night lights are readily available. Some parents have found that black-out blinds or a blanket at the window helps, especially in the summer when light from outside may convince your child that it's time to play. You could also try moving the cot or bed into a recess, or moving your child to a different room altogether.

Wrap more Snugly

Many cultures prevent free-limb movement as a way of soothing babies and encouraging them to relax. Some Western parents may feel that this is unnatural or even cruel. Yet babies tend to fall asleep or become quietly alert when they are snuggled tightly. Such babies also seem to cry less, sleep more, have a slower heartbeat and breathe more regularly.

In cultures where swaddling is the norm, as with the Navajo Indians, the babies are tightly wrapped and placed vertically on a 'cradleboard'. The mother takes her baby wherever she goes, so he can watch her at work and she can talk to him. Several times a day she removes him from the cradleboard just so she can cuddle him. Babies seem to like it, maybe because they get handled more often, and maybe because they're more involved in family life. In fact, babies brought up on cradleboards tend to develop physically slightly ahead of Western babies.

In many other cultures including some South American Indians – the Yequana from Venezuela, and the Peruvian Nunoa Quecha – babies are carried from birth until about a year, either on the hip or in a sling. The difficulties with this approach for most Western women are that we tend not to live in extended families where there is always someone to hold the baby, that our paid work and our domestic lives are usually separate, and that women tend not to live such physically active lives, so that carrying a child until he is one is hard work.

Some parents, however, manage to approximate to this sort of life by using a combination of slings or backpacks, staying home and slowing their lives down.

> I changed my general approach to Thomas at five months old. This was because he had seemed to cry a lot during the day all of a sudden. I had developed a sore back moving him from room to room in his baby seat. I read the book *The Continuum Concept* by Jean Leidloff. That very afternoon I started to carry him around with me to see how I did various tasks. All of a sudden my back felt better, even though I was holding him a lot and he was happy again.
>
> **Sarah**

Touch

Many babies find a massage very soothing, and may fall asleep during or immediately after one. This sleep period is often in addition to the normal sleep your baby takes. The earlier you start massaging your baby, the better. By the time he is crawling, your baby may just crawl away. You can learn a technique through a book or a video but attending a class run by a qualified baby masseur is best as the books can't give you feedback about how you're doing and the baby on the video might like a different touch to your baby. Massage will teach your baby how to let go of tension and will help you to get closer to him. It's a particularly good skill for a new dad to learn.

Massage teaches a parent to respond to their individual child. A full-body massage may take 20 minutes. If you spend that long with your baby, you learn a lot of his likes and dislikes. Massage also has physical benefits: it improves the circulation, deepens and regulates the breathing, increases the level of oxygen in the bloodstream (which leads to deeper sleep), promotes muscle tone and helps with the development of the nervous system by stimulating areas that are furthest from the brain. Massage introduces your baby to his body.

To find out about baby massage classes in your area, contact the International Association of Infant Massage, see page 151.

Company

Some babies seem to need company to be able to fall asleep. Some parents are happy to remain with their baby until he sleeps. Others stay with their baby because they see no option, or fight a running battle up and down the stairs each evening. Some parents find that putting their baby to sleep in the same room as a sibling helps.

Daniel just wanted company. I was lying down in the evening with him for two hours at a time, and then as soon as he was asleep I was collapsing into bed myself. I was really low. Then a friend said to put him in with Georgia, his older sister. It was amazing, within about two weeks he'd stopped calling out and Georgia never woke up, although once or twice since then we have found him in her bed when we go in in the morning.

For some parents, sleeping with their baby solves some problems and creates others:

> Until Hannah was 15 months old she spent the nights in our bed so she could nurse whenever she wanted with the minimum disruption as she woke four or five times a night. But she took over our bed by lying across it, I frequently ended up sleeping curled up in a quarter of the bed next to my husband's feet! So when she was 15 months old we put a mattress on the floor of her bedroom so when she woke I could lie down with her and she could stay in her own bed.

Dawn, mother of Rebecca, six, Hannah, four, and Lucy, 18 months

Music and Movement

Many young babies are soothed by sound and movement – continuous, rhythmic sounds and movement work best. You could try womb music (tape available from NCT Maternity Sales website, see page 152), or a vacuum cleaner, although this option may be less appealing at night. From a few months before he is born your baby is able to hear sounds outside your body. Some mothers find that songs they sing or music they play at this time have a particularly calming effect on their baby once he is born.

Richard, father of Hannah, aged nine months, found that loud and insistent music rapidly stopped her crying at night:

> I used to rock her while I was walking up and down. It was incredibly boring so I put on some loud music and the insistence of the rhythm overwhelmed her senses and she went to sleep. I think it was Verdi's Rigoletto, and some Stephen Stills that were the most effective. But then she's always had great taste in music – just like her father!

Naturally, the effect isn't always so immediate, which is probably why so many traditional folk songs have at least a dozen verses.

Many babies are soothed by travelling in a car, but all too often wake as soon as the engine stops. This can be an expensive, time-consuming and less than 'green' way to get your baby to sleep regularly, although many families resort to it in desperation.

Simon used to take Rachael out in the car in the evening, it was easier than listening to her cry. She was fine when the car was moving. But as soon as he stopped she'd wake, unless he drove for long enough so that she was really deeply asleep. But even then it was almost impossible to transfer her, still asleep, into her cot, because the car was parked so far from the front door. But at least I had a break.

Simon and Julie, parents of Rachael and Sylvie

If your baby needs a lot of rocking, more than your back can bear or you have time for, you might want to consider buying a swinging cradle which you push by hand and which your baby can use from birth to about four months. Alternatively a baby swing, suitable for babies from four to nine months, will rock him for 15 minutes at a time when wound up. See page 152 for suppliers. Homoeopathy may also help the baby who likes a lot of motion.

Homoeopathy

It's unlikely that you can cure a sleep problem with homoeopathy alone, but it may calm your child enough so that other solutions work. And even if it doesn't work, it will have done no harm. As with all homoeopathic remedies, the remedies for sleep disruptions treat the person rather than the symptoms. Your sleepless baby may fit one of two common temperaments, and may be helped by over-the-counter homoeopathic remedies. You may want to consult a homoeopath; the address of the British Homoeopathic Association is on page 151.

Try pulsatilla to calm your baby when he seems to need to be with you to sleep but wakes or cries as soon as you move away. This is the one for you when you want to stop playing musical beds.

Try chamomilla when your baby is crotchety or irritable, when he wants you not only to be with him but to move as well. It's certainly a much greener alternative to driving your baby around in the car to get him to sleep. Chamomilla is better known as the active ingredient in homoeopathic teething granules for use when your baby is teething and irritable with it.

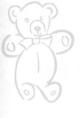

9

Coping with Feelings, Gaining Support

I can remember thinking how easy it would be to smash his head against a wall when he was six to 12 months.

Diana

We live by a river and there were times I used to think that if I just let go of the pram I could go home and have some sleep. I was going to bed at 8pm. My husband and I had no relationship.

Amanda, mother of Ben, aged five months

Sleeping problems can tear families apart – especially when they are severe or long lasting. In families where the stress level is already high, like those in which there is a child with a disability, or where there are relationship problems or money or housing problems, the addition of sleep problems can make the stress almost intolerable.

Your Feelings for your Baby

Sometimes the strength of your feelings can shock you. Kim, mother of three-year-old Rowan, who still wakes frequently at night, says:

> This sleep problem has brought out the worst in me at times – I admit to having hated my daughter. I get frustrated because I have really tried to solve this problem. You love your children so much and you give so much of yourself to them that it becomes painful to see them as little horrors.

Parents whose children do not settle themselves back to sleep at night can suffer from the double whammy of sleep loss and feelings of failure. Not only does the sleep loss affect your ability to do everyday tasks, but it can also leave you questioning your abilities as a parent. You can end up feeling stressed and lacking in self-confidence (Wolson *et al.*, 1992).

> Laura didn't go through the night until she was ten months, and that was just a one-off. It was absolutely exhausting. I ended up with postnatal depression. I was like a zombie, but I don't think that that was the depression, I think it was just that I couldn't sleep.

Sally, mother of Laura and Annie

> All my friend's babies slept 12 hours and I felt a real failure.

Karen, mother of David

You may also feel angry, extremely anxious, depressed, exhausted, murderous, inadequate, desperate, resentful or helpless. Jenny felt pretty much all of these things about Owen:

> I have an absolute nightmare child who won't sleep for more than one-and-a-half hours day or night. At six-and-a-half months he needs me right next to him. You want to talk about resentful? I'm telling you I'm really resentful. I can't cope with how I feel. At times I've had to stop myself hurting him. I've done some awful things to him. I've bitten his fingers when he's stuffed them in my mouth, I've screamed at him, I've slapped his legs in the middle of the night, I've shaken him to make him cry in the middle of the night. I do have a temper, I know I have a temper and ... and ... we should all be asleep.

Fiona also got to breaking point:

> Phoebe was 13 months old and had never slept longer than about two hours at a time and did not sleep during the day. I had become very run down and could no longer cope with the day-to-day ups and downs of being a mother. I spent my hours alone with her crying and screaming at the slightest thing. I shook her and handled her roughly and frequently had to leave the room in order not to hurt her.

If you feel that you may injure your baby, put him down – gently – and leave the room. He is safer crying on his own than he is with you right now. Talk to someone you can trust or do something else for five minutes until you feel calmer. Shaking a baby is the single largest cause of infant death in Britain today. It won't help him to sleep and it won't help you feel better, but it may cause serious damage to him or even kill him. When you feel like this, try not to add to these powerful emotions by feeling bad about such feelings, or trying to hide them. Admit that you feel this way now; most parents get to this pitch at some point. Try to believe that it won't always be like this.

Feelings of frustration that nothing works or at the amount of control your baby exerts over you are common. Jane and David, parents of Nicholas, Adam and George, found that their frustration and tension eased after they accepted that Nicholas wanted to share their bed.

Looking back, I think that our need to get, especially the first baby, to sleep was linked to a struggle to accept the change in our lives – to somehow reclaim time alone, without the baby. Once we came to accept him and subsequent children more, then the babies' failure to sleep when we wanted them to became less of a problem.

Feelings like these can eat away at you. Find someone to talk to who will just listen, without offering you any advice. Sometimes there is nothing separating the sleeping patterns of one family from another – the babies are both difficult to settle in the evening, wake and cry the same number of times in the night, and take just as long to fall asleep again. What's different is the emotions that the waking evokes. How you feel about it is as much a part of the problem as what happens in the middle of the night. Once you can accept and face your feelings, they may not torture you so much and you can concentrate on accepting or changing the behaviour that leaves you feeling this way.

Finding Support

Sleeping problems are easier to tackle when you feel supported in your choices. Most parents start by talking to their partner. Often you think you know what your partner feels or expects, and your partner thinks he knows you too. Often you're right. But where there is tension or things don't feel right, it's imperative that you sit down and talk about it. Naturally, now that you have a baby there's no time for talking. If only you didn't have the baby you could find time to sit and talk about the baby ... But all relationships – the good, the bad and the downright wobbly – are tested by the arrival of a baby. A baby who doesn't sleep compounds the problem. Talking is one of the best ways to remain in touch with your partner. So, book a slot and stick to it.

> Natashia and I used to have our baths together because it meant I was ready for bed when she was. One night Alan came home early and we were already in the bath and he just took off his suit and got in with us. We couldn't stop laughing, and it was freezing, because no-one could lie down and we couldn't have the water too hot because of Natashia, but we really had a good talk about how things were.

Carol and Alan, parents of Natashia and Luke

Sharing the Load

> We've been through periods where my husband and I have been at each other's throats, just because I was tired.

Kim, mother of Rowan and Lloyd

Many women say they have to get up to their baby at night because their partner has a responsible job.

Researchers have discovered what most exhausted women already knew: that tiredness can seriously impair your relationship with your baby and with your other children. And it can strain your relationship with your partner, sometimes terminally. So tell me, who has a responsible job?

- Do things as parents for your baby, rather than just taking turns
- Ask your partner to cuddle you as you feed the baby
- Be patient with each other as you learn what works
- Try not to give each other too many pointers, make your own way with your baby
- Affirm each other's growing skills: when things go well, describe what happened ('You picked her up and she stopped crying'). When things go badly, make your suggestions gently ('Sometimes she seems to like her back rubbed').

If your relationship is suffering from lack of sleep, take heart; researchers have discovered that when children do start to sleep better, their parents feel less depressed in themselves and happier in their marriages or partnerships (Durant and Mindell, 1990). But not all partnerships weather the storm.

Victoria's relationship with her husband, Dave, has never been the same since Helena was born:

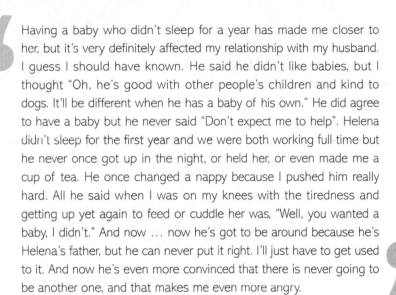

Having a baby who didn't sleep for a year has made me closer to her, but it's very definitely affected my relationship with my husband. I guess I should have known. He said he didn't like babies, but I thought "Oh, he's good with other people's children and kind to dogs. It'll be different when he has a baby of his own." He did agree to have a baby but he never said "Don't expect me to help". Helena didn't sleep for the first year and we were both working full-time but he never once got up in the night, or held her, or even made me a cup of tea. He once changed a nappy because I pushed him really hard. All he said when I was on my knees with the tiredness and getting up yet again to feed or cuddle her was, "Well, you wanted a baby, I didn't." And now ... now he's got to be around because he's Helena's father, but he can never put it right. I'll just have to get used to it. And now he's even more convinced that there is never going to be another one, and that makes me even more angry.

Sorting out a fair split can be tricky. For example, if you need a solid ten hours and your partner is fine on the standard eight, then maybe your partner should get up more often, even if it means that you both end up with less sleep than you'd like. Alternatively, if you have serious difficulty going back to sleep once you're woken, then maybe one of you will need to move out of the parental bed and leave your partner to it.

 Simon decided to sleep elsewhere, while William was in our bed, because he developed ME. In a way, although it meant I had to do everything on my own it was something positive – to have William with me while Simon was ill.

Ann

Some parents work out a 'one night on, one night off' system so that they know they can sleep well every other night; others take shifts through the night. Just remember that six hours of unbroken sleep leaves you better rested than eight hours of broken sleep. Most of us have entered the 'I'm more tired than you' competition more than once, but it's a competition that no one wins.

Harriet, who tried and succeeded with what she calls the 'reassurance principle', found that her husband's support was invaluable:

Mostly we experienced it as a shared frustration. It was the focus of different ideas about children and the differences led to some resentment and frustration at times. At others the shared exhaustion engendered a sort of Dunkirk spirit!

Harriet, mother of Nicholas, 11, Adam, nine, and George, six

Emily slept from 11pm to 3am from birth without a feed but at six weeks we decided we wanted our evenings back. So, using Jo Douglas and Naomi Richman's book, *My Child Won't Sleep* we decided to leave her alone when she had been fed and changed and was comfortable and needed nothing else. We would go in every five minutes and stay with her until her crying subsided, and she was at the sobbing stage, and then leave. Each night we brought back bedtime by 10 minutes until it reached 8pm and she slept through for eleven hours with one feed at 11pm. Now at ten-and-a-half months she goes down at 7pm and sleeps right through. In the night when she woke I used the trick of counting from 100 back to one before I'd go in to her. More often than not, she went back to sleep again. A couple of times we just let her scream herself to sleep – but unless Will had been there I couldn't have done it.

But failing such equality, having a sleeping partner in the business of cracking a sleep problem improves your chances of success. Even if you are the one lumbering back and forth between your room and your baby's or lying pinned to the bed by the weight of your child's head on your chest, it is immeasurably helpful to know that the person sleeping warm and soundly beside you or on the sofa downstairs agrees with what you're doing.

Asking for Support when you're a Lone Parent

- Invite a friend or your mum to stay just so that you can have a break for a night or for those first few long nights when you start a new routine
- Start the routine on your own on a Friday night and ask your friend to look after your baby on Saturday and Sunday afternoon so that you can sleep
- Swap your baby with a friend's baby for one night a week. It can work – the babies may sleep and so will you

Having a sleepless baby can make you feel isolated, especially if you are a lone parent. Take care of yourself. Try to arrange for someone to visit or phone you each day, even if you can't get out yourself. When you're feeling stronger, make use of parent and toddler groups (your local library will have a list), or contact your local branch of the National Childbirth Trust or Meet-A-Mum, who can put you in touch with other parents. The addresses of these organizations are on pages 157 and 149.

Handling Advice

It's one of the unwritten rules of parenthood that anyone who has a sleep problem must be surrounded by friends and family, all of whom know how to cure it and are willing to tell you at great length. Fiona demonstrates the rule:

Wherever I went, without fail, the first question anyone asked was "Is she good?" Now everyone knows that they did not want a moral judgement on the state of Phoebe's tiny baby soul. Translated, this question actually means "Does she sleep a lot and cry a little?" And naturally I had to reply "No". It hurt me that to all intents and purposes I was telling people that my baby was bad. I began to rebel. Why, in our society, is good equated with sleeping and keeping quiet? So when asked, I would say, "Her character is perfect, it is only her sleeping pattern which is erratic."

As Phoebe grew, the question changed slightly. It was still the first thing anyone asked, but had developed into "Has she slept through the night yet?" This did not just mean total coma from 8am until 8pm, it had to be in her own room without any lullabies or hands being held or even dummy to suck (not that she liked them anyway). Then the advice started, whether we asked for it or not: "Don't pick her up every time she cries, you're spoiling her"; "You've got to get her into a proper routine"; "You're not still breastfeeding that child are you?", "Give her a bottle last thing at night"; "She's a big baby, she needs some solids in her tummy"; "She's using you as a dummy"; "Leave her to cry …", "Leave her to cry …", "Leave her to cry …" And the most offensive of all: "If you gave her to me for a couple of nights I'd have the little madam sorted out, I can tell you".

You're the expert on your baby. Talk to as many people as possible about what works for them, but remember that they aren't looking after your baby and they aren't you. Your solution for your family's sleep problem needs to sit comfortably with the way you like to handle things. If you do anything else, it won't work for you.

 My mother in law said: "Leave that baby to cry". But we didn't do it while she was there, we wanted to do it ourselves. As soon as she left, we tried it – and it worked.

Liz, mother of four

However, if you do want to make some changes there is a lot of support available outside the family. An appointment with your GP or health visitor is often the first port of call. Talk to them about your plans. Both these health professionals will offer you common-sense advice about getting your child to sleep, or refer you to a local sleep clinic. Your GP will also be able to advise you, or refer you elsewhere if you think your baby may be waking in pain or is allergic. Brief assessment visits in hospital are available, but rare.

 Going into hospital for Ben's sleeping problem when he was four months old was the worst thing I'd ever done and the best thing. In the night the nurses did the comforting, and he learnt to do what we couldn't show him how to. (From birth he wanted feeding every two hours, and my husband and I were exhausted. I'd been to a sleep clinic, but I wasn't able to do the programme at home – I couldn't tolerate hearing him cry, I would just go in and feed him, or my husband would go in and stay with him until he went to sleep.) I felt so guilty. I was leaving him to cry with a complete stranger. But we were able to catch up on a bit of sleep and he got the idea of what was going to happen. He's a lot happier now because he has enough sleep.

Amanda and Michael, parents of Ben, aged five months

If the sleeping problem is severe and you are at the end of your tether, your GP may prescribe drugs for your baby.

Drugs

Most doctors only prescribe sleeping drugs to babies when the problems are severe, have gone on for a long time and you are close to breaking point. This is because sleeping drugs do not solve sleeping problems. They will only offer you a few nights' respite. Your doctor will probably only prescribe drugs sufficient for two or three nights, and no more than two weeks at the outside.

The two most commonly prescribed sleeping drugs are trimeprazine, under the brand name of Vallergan, and promethazine, which is sold as Phenergan. However, your doctor may be reluctant to prescribe either of these as they are not recommended for use with babies under two.

It is important that you give your baby the stated dose, rather than try a small amount first, as sleeping drugs have a hyperactive effect at low doses, and your baby may simply stay awake longer than usual. Some parents find that a drug prescription is reassuring. It says that their problem is serious and that if they can't cope, there is something they can do. Often parents then decide to treat the problem another way. A lot of sleeping drugs are prescribed and never used.

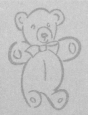 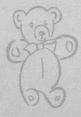 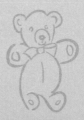 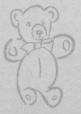

When you get to the stage where you need to use drugs you are desperate, you'll try anything. You've got to get some sleep. I was feeding James every two hours night and day, and because he was a slow feeder it took me an hour each time. I slept for an hour and fed for an hour. Because he was my first, I was expecting it to be a wonder drug – it wasn't. First of all I was given the wrong dose of Phenergan and it made him hyperactive. Then I was prescribed Vallergan which knocked him out and gave me more than two hours at a time. But it didn't break the habit. It didn't solve my problems. He was tired in the mornings and a bit dopey in the day, and then of course, he wasn't tired enough to have an afternoon nap until late, and by bedtime he wasn't tired enough to sleep and you're not supposed to give it to them until they wake for the first time in the evening.

Teresa, mother of James, nine, Emma, six, and Mark, four

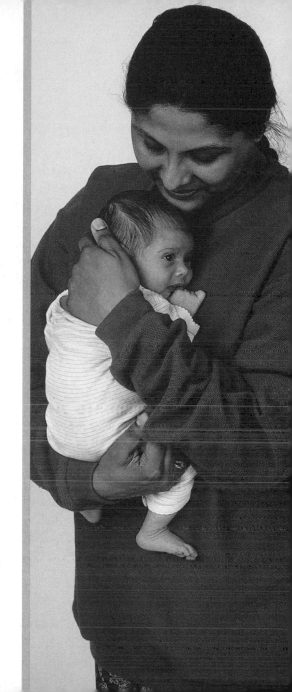

Sleep Therapy

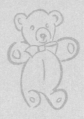

Sleep Clinics

Sleep clinics are groups run by health visitors and occasionally other health professionals too. After an initial session in which you describe your baby's sleep habits, you will usually be asked to complete a sleep diary for a couple of weeks before you begin a programme. Nearly all sleep clinics will suggest a peaceful and predictable bedtime routine, followed by a form of behaviour modification – usually either controlled crying or gradual withdrawal. Most sleep clinics assume that you would like your child to go to sleep on his own in his own bed. Some research suggests that more than 80% of parents who join groups led by health professionals can successfully stop a sleep problem. For more information, ask your health visitor or GP about your local sleep clinic.

One-to-One Sessions with a Sleep Therapist

Sleep therapists are a rare breed, but where they can be found they are available privately and occasionally by referral from your GP. Your health visitor or GP may have contact details. Or ask your friends. Sometimes you will see a team of health professionals. A sleep therapist will see you, your partner and your baby for one or more sessions and will discuss ways to solve your sleep problems. Most of them include behaviour management plans as part of their solution. Some sleep therapists claim 100% success when parents attend weekly.

Brief Psychoanalytic Therapy

This is available at a few places round the country. It is a radically different approach to sleeping problems. Over four or five sessions, a child psychotherapist will help you to explore the boundaries within your family, and support you while you work towards letting your child sleep. The emphasis of the sessions is not on practical plans but on understanding how aspects of your past and present – grief, separation, loss – can hamper your ability to let your baby go (see page 150 for contact details).

Child and Family Consultation Clinics (CFCC)
(formerly known as Child Guidance)

These clinics offer a similar service to the brief psychoanalytic therapy above, with the added advantage that there are more CFCCs around the country. Your GP may refer you to a child and family consultation clinic if your sleeping problem is part of a more general problem with relationships in your family.

Self Help

Some parents set up their own support group. This is a particularly good idea if you don't want to leave your baby to sleep alone. Whatever you opt for, the important thing is to find yourself someone who listens well, is available in times of crisis and can support your choices.

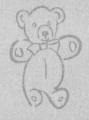

10

Alternative Help

Just occasionally a sleep problem may be the result of pain. Babies express pain in many different ways including being clingy, excessive sucking and screaming when laid down flat (if your baby is in pain he may prefer to sleep in a semi-upright position). If your baby has any of these symptoms, consult your GP. Some parents have found that an alternative treatment has unearthed the root cause of their baby's sleep problem.

Hyperactivity and Allergic Reactions

Hyperactive children have difficulty sleeping and often wake early. There is a lot of controversy about the causes of hyperactivity. Some doctors claim that diet is at the root of the problem and some that diet is only a small part of the answer.

An allergic reaction to food and additives, or to materials, washing powder or dust, can keep your child awake in many ways, depending on the symptoms that it causes. Your child may have frequent ear or chest infections, be hyperactive or cry, have an abnormal thirst and/or a poor appetite, have eczema, dribble, head bang or rock his cot excessively. None of these symptoms conclusively proves that your child has an allergy; but if several of them occur continuously, you might consider an allergy test. An allergy clinic will test your child on an enormous array of known allergens: foods, fabrics, perfumes, dust and hair to name a few. But you may have to pay. Your health visitor or GP will have details of services in your area, or contact the Hyperactive Children's Support Group (address on page 151).

The most likely causes of food-related allergies are dairy products, sugar and chocolate, additives (particularly tartrazine or E102), oranges, orange juice and eggs.

Anna had undiagnosed allergic reactions as her mother, Janet, remembers:

Anna had colic when she was little, and I used to sit downstairs until 2am to stop her sister waking up. When she went onto solids, the colic got worse. She became constipated and would only poo every four to five days. When she did poo it was really painful for her and she'd cry out and hold on to it. I used to sit in the bathroom for an hour at a time, just waiting. The night after she pooed she would sleep through the night, but every other night she would shout in her sleep and go rigid.

At 22 months she was allergy tested. She is allergic to potatoes, rice, tomatoes, egg and peanuts. If you think what all the baby food is made up of, it's not surprising weaning made her worse. We took her off all the foods she is allergic to and that night she became hyperactive – asking for all sorts of foods and tearing the wallpaper border off her wall. She still only poos every two or three days because she's used to it hurting her, but her sleep is a lot better – although now I have to stop her going to bed with a bottle, a habit that we got into when the doctor told me to help her constipation by giving her more fluids – the only advice he ever gave me.

Acupuncture

One form of acupuncture identifies four different energy states – hot, cold, delicate and frightened. Your baby may have elements of any or all of these states. The hot baby wakes and wants to play in the middle of the night. The cold baby, whose mother may have had a lot of drugs at birth, or who may have been exposed to draughts at birth, arches his back, has blue tinges to the lips and seems to have pain around his middle. The delicate baby is often the child of older parents who, in the wisdom of Chinese medicine, will have less useful energy than younger parents. This baby may want to eat or be comforted, to be nurtured or massaged. The frightened baby is not easily soothed, but may be helped by a night light.

Food is also seen as giving different energy states which produce hot or cold insomnia symptoms. So, a therapist would help your child to eat towards the opposite of what they are, without tipping the scales too far in the opposite direction.

Acupuncture Tips

Acupuncturists divide food into groups – hot, warm, cool and cold.

A food's heat is part of the food itself, whether straight from the fridge or out of the oven. They also believe that foods in the cold group can cause colic: food like bananas and yoghurt, which are often some of the earliest solids given to babies. So, if your baby suffers from colic, keep him off the bananas and yoghurt for a week. It may just help.

Chinese acupuncturists also use a range of different tools including needles, massage, small suction cups and low-level lasers to stimulate energy flow. If needles are used, then the practitioner will pop them in and out very quickly so that your baby does not have to stay still for a long time. There may be a little soreness and a few tears, but these are quickly over. Parents often worry more about the needles than their child. You should see results after about four sessions.

Although treatments can be expensive, many therapists operate concessionary sliding scales. Acupuncture may also be available free on the NHS with a referral from your GP. Some private health schemes will also pay for acupuncture treatments. Check your policy to find out.

Enza and Claudio took Valentina to see an acupuncturist when she was 16 months old:

> Valentina had no rhythm, no pattern. Sometimes she would sleep in the day, sometimes at night. Very rarely she slept for five or six hours. Her feeding was all over the place as well, so I couldn't stop breastfeeding her until after the treatment. Sometimes she would wake in the night to play and then sleep better in the day. At the first session the acupuncturist asked a lot of questions, particularly about the birth – I had a caesarean, and that was part of the problem. At the first session Valentina had some laser treatment. But after that she had the needles, which went in for a fraction of a second. Somehow I knew it would be the needles that worked best, and it was. Since the treatment she has slept quite well even when she was teething.
>
> A lot of it was to do with diet. I had to cut right down on dairy products, and now she seems to prefer soya milk. The acupuncturists said she had a lot of heat. She would always throw the covers off from the moment she was born, but since the treatment that's all gone. Her character's still the same but I think she is calmer. Now she sleeps for seven hours without waking up, but that doesn't mean that she won't go back to sleep again, I just give her a drink of water and she goes back to sleep. I would recommend anyone to try acupuncture.

See page 150 for details of how to contact a registered acupuncturist trained to work with children. And do make sure that your acupuncturist is registered as there is currently no legislation to prevent anyone setting themselves up as an acupuncturist.

Cranial Osteopathy

Cranial osteopathy is based on the idea that pregnancy and birth are traumatic times for babies. Each baby has the ability to unwind from that trauma, but some get stuck. The trauma is then held and expressed in their bodies. Sleep disturbance can be one expression of this trauma.

With new-born babies it is possible for a therapist to just lay his hands on the skull and for there to be a change within minutes.

Most cranial osteopaths work with the baby while he is being held by his parents. This allows the baby to feel secure with the changes that occur and for the parents to see the baby differently. This is especially useful where your relationship with your baby has been strained by a lack of sleep.

The therapist will usually begin by placing his hands on your baby's head to tune in to the restrictions he is experiencing, although he could move to any part of the baby's body where he senses restrictions. There will be nothing for you to see except for a change in the baby, as the therapist does not physically manipulate your baby. Therapists describe what they do as tuning in and listening to the baby and then allowing the baby to use his natural healing ability to move to a place of ease.

The average baby needs between two and five weekly sessions, with a check-up later. See the information section on page 151 for details on how to contact a registered therapist near you.

Harry, my second, would never sleep properly. I had a normal delivery, but a very quick second stage and his head was very bruised. I never had any trouble putting him in his cot in the evening, it was the waking up in the night and screaming as though he had his fingers caught in the door. At 11 months I got to absolute despair. After the first six weeks he never slept in the day, the best I ever got was 20 minutes. He'd wake up five or six times a night and all he'd want to do was feed.

He absolutely refused to take a bottle. I tried to stop feeding him, but day and night all he wanted to do was feed and Oliver, my eldest, would play me up as soon as I started feeding in the day. At 11 months I rang my health visitor. I said "I can't even think straight, I just don't know what to do." She could hear I was desperate and she came to see me. She told me about sleep therapy and about cranial osteopathy. I was really worried about the sleep therapy group because I thought they were going to give us such a hard time, but actually they were very sympathetic. They said, "How do you work your day?" and "How do you deal with Harry at night?" and then they said, "You're not doing anything wrong."

Well, we tried the controlled crying technique and the longest he cried was for five-and-a-half hours. After that I went in and said "You've won." Then we got a cancelled appointment with the cranial osteopath. He said, "Yes, we can help you and you'll have to come back three or four times." He told us that Harry had a strain on the front of his skull. I had to imagine it was like an elastic band from his jaw to the top of his head.

The night after the first treatment my husband went in and checked on him and he said he was sleeping in a baby pose, with his hands up by his head, not the fetal position. He was relaxed for the first time. After three treatments he slept through. He's not the perfect sleeper, he still wakes up once a night but the turning point was when he started to call for me instead of scream. The cranial osteopathy changed our lives.

Debbie

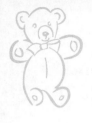

11

Behaviour Management

I'm definitely one for leaving them to cry – it's definitely the only way to do it.

Liz, mother of four

I've always refused to leave my baby to cry, thinking this cruel and unnecessary – especially when young, when they need comfort.

Emily, mother of Imogen, aged 13 months

Leaving a baby to cry is an emotive phrase. Behaviour management, sensitively handled, is less about leaving your baby to cry and more about leaving him to sleep. It means giving your baby the chance to fall asleep alone, by putting him down sleepy but awake. Most behaviour management programmes involve returning to your baby at pre-determined intervals to reassure him and yourself that everything is alright.

- *Cueing* Helping your baby to learn a new behaviour by providing him with the same cues regularly. For example, you provide a regular bedtime routine for your baby, so that he knows when it's time for sleep (see page 28 for more on routines).
- *Extinction* You stop rewarding your baby for the behaviour you don't like. Babies find an amazing array of activities rewarding. Naturally, nearly all babies enjoy a cuddle, a song, a story, a drink, a smile, a carry, a video, or any other nurturing, companionable activity. But your baby might also find it rewarding when you yell or shout – he won't find it pleasant but it is attention, and any sort of attention is rewarding.
- *Reinforcement* You reward or praise your baby when he does things the new way. For example, using a star chart (see page 126 on star charts), or telling him how pleased you are that he stayed in bed/slept all night/got up at 7am instead of 5am.
- *Shaping* Changing your behaviour and his gradually. For example, bringing bedtime ten minutes earlier each night or giving him less and less attention as he falls asleep each night.

You can use the principles of behaviour management to help your baby improve a whole range of sleep problems, and it works for all sorts of children, of all ages, although you may want to try one of the slower approaches if your baby is experiencing separation anxiety (see Chapter 6).

The programme works best when you believe that

- it is in everyone's best interests
- this is the best way to do it

- you and your baby can manage it, and
- you feel supported in your choices.

It doesn't work for everyone.

> We tried letting Rhian cry and it didn't work at all. There was no improvement. She would cry for one-and-a-half hours every night and fall asleep with exhaustion. We thought it wasn't fair. She started to whimper when she saw her cot during the day. So it doesn't always work.

Dilys and Mick

But it does work for many others.

> The book says it works within a week, but for myself and two friends our children were sleeping through the night sooner. The first night of the programme was the worst. This harsher treatment has not caused our second child to be less confident as some books and people suggest. She is very calm, whereas my first makes mountains out of mole-hills.

Brenda and Dave, parents of Mark and Esme

How to do it

Keep a sleep diary for a week before you make any changes so that you can see where the problems and the patterns occur. Choose a week when no one is ill and nothing out of the ordinary is planned. Keep the diary and a pen next to your bed, so you can jot things down as they happen. Make a note of what the whole family did, where and when. Sometimes siblings can make a difference to your baby's sleep pattern. Copy the chart opposite or make your own.

> When we were having problems getting Kate to sleep through, my husband suggested I keep a sleep diary. You get in a blur — it just seems to get things in perspective.

Tessa and Alan, parents of Jack, three, and Kate, two

Sleep Diary

Child's name: Child's age: Week number:

	Fri	Sat	Sun	Mon	Tue	Wed	Thur
Time woke in the morning Mood on waking What did you do?							
Time and length of naps in the day							
Time and length of meals in the day							
Time started preparing for bed Any problems here? What did you do?							
Time went to bed at night, and where? How long did your child take to settle? What did you do?							
Time went to sleep							
Times and length of waking at night Total time awake What did you do?							

Use your sleep diary to identify the problem areas: needing you to be there when he falls asleep in the evening or at night; elongated bedtimes; night waking; night feeds; late bedtimes and early mornings. This chapter deals with night waking and settling in the evening; the following chapter deals with moving the time at which your child sleeps. If you're still feeding at night, have a look at Chapter 5 as well.

When you're ready to start your new routine pick a time to do it. Some parents find that it's better to do it in the day first, when they have more energy. Others find that it works better to concentrate on the evening and night first and let the day fall into place. The weekend is often a good time to start so that you can catch up on the sleep you lose more easily. Keep a sleep diary while you are using the new routine. It will show you where you are making progress and where you may need to make more changes. If you are following one of the programmes with the support of a health professional or friend, your sleep diary will probably help them to see what is going on as well.

Devise and stick to a simple and relaxed pre-bedtime routine (see Chapter 3 for ideas about routines). Once you've tucked your child into bed and kissed him goodnight, you have four options.

Option 1: Cold Turkey

If you want to achieve some results quickly, leave your child to sleep and do not go back at all. You may have to bear a lot of crying, but it is likely that after the first few days your child will go to sleep easily on his own. However, this approach often fails because it is too traumatic for parents and babies alike. Leaving your child to sleep like this can be quite shocking for both of you, especially when your previous goodbyes have been long.

> Leaving Thomas to cry from six weeks did work over a couple of months and not feeding him until 4am or later gradually encouraged him not to bother waking.

Jane

Option 2: Controlled Crying

Alternatively, leave your baby to sleep but return every so often to reassure yourself and him.

After the bedtime routine on the first night, stay out of sight for five minutes; if he is still crying after this time, return and reassure him that you are still there. If he is standing up, lay him down; if he is still lying down, gently stroke him. Then leave. This time wait for ten minutes; if he is still crying and shows no signs of quietening, go in again and repeat what you said before. The next time leave it for 15 minutes. On the first night, leave a maximum of 15 minutes between all subsequent visits. The whole procedure may take anything between two or three hours the first night. Older children usually take longer and tiny babies less time.

On the second night, wait for ten minutes before you go to reassure him for the first time, and then 15 and then a maximum of 20 for all successive visits. This time the total time until he sleeps should be shorter. On subsequent nights increase the waiting times by five minutes.

Leave your baby to go to sleep for this many minutes before you return to reassure him briefly. There's nothing magical about these timings. Decide what you and your baby can manage and stick to it.

Night	first check	second check	third check	subsequent checks
1	5	10	15	15
2	10	15	20	20
3	15	20	25	25
4	20	25	30	30
5	25	30	35	35
6	30	35	40	40
7	35	40	45	45 and so on.

Some parents like to look their child straight in the eye and say something like 'Go to sleep now'; others prefer to deliberately avoid their child's gaze and just pat their child's back or lay him down again, or you could try the approach on page 21. It's up to you. The important thing is to do the same thing on each occasion, and make it simple and minimal. Do not give him anything that he cannot get on his own. You want him to be able to go to sleep without needing you. So don't offer a bottle or a cuddle or a song. It is important to sound and behave confidently. Your confidence is your child's security.

Karen and Phil tried the checking approach with David for three and a half months of disturbed nights before they realized that they had been doing it wrong:

> We used to go in to David three or four times a night, using the controlled crying technique each time. But it just didn't seem to work – he kept on waking up. We were just so tired. I'd got to the point where I really hated him. I thought, "I've made a big mistake having children at all."
>
> It was only after we'd been battling with it for three and a half months that I read somewhere that we shouldn't be giving him a bottle whenever he woke, because he would wake up just to get it. I'd been giving him one because I just hadn't realized that there comes a time when babies don't need something at night. So we stopped the bottle, it was only water, and within two nights he slept through. Only for six hours, but it was wonderful. It really works, you just have to do it properly.

If he calms down significantly while you are out of the room, do not go back in to him. A visit from you at this point may make him start all over again. Check on him once he is finally asleep, if you want to, but leave it at least half an hour so that you can be sure he is deeply asleep.

Be prepared for a test time on the third, fourth or fifth night. Your baby has understood that this is the new routine and is making one last-ditch attempt to get things back to where they were and his cries may be longer and more bitter than before. Once this long night is over you should be almost there, although for some people the process is longer.

> I did the five-minute routine suggested by the counsellor. She said it would solve the problem in six weeks. It actually took three months to do. We got it down to one night waking – I could live with that. It is painful. They can cry for a long time if you keep going back. I wrote down everything that happened – how I felt, what I did. It allowed me to see how things had changed. I did some sewing or the ironing so that I didn't feel so resentful when she kept going for two hours.

Kim, mother of Rowan and Lloyd

Option 3: the Kissing Game

Try this procedure if your child appears anxious at bedtime or needy in the day or if you don't feel right leaving him alone to sleep. It is particularly suitable for children between six months and two years, but it can be used for pre-schoolers too.

After a relaxed bedtime routine, kiss your baby goodnight, and promise to return in a minute to give another kiss. In fact, you should return almost immediately to give another kiss, take a few steps away and then another kiss, put away something in the room and then kiss again, pop outside for a few seconds and then another kiss, and so on. So long as your child is lying down with his head on the pillow, or on the cot mattress, he gets more kisses, but no more chat, cuddles, stories, plays or drinks. Just kisses until he is asleep. Think of yourself as being on a piece of elastic – bobbing back and forth to your child.

If your child jumps out of bed, keep it light. Say something like 'Come on now, you know the deal, into bed and I'll give you a kiss.' Then help him back to bed. Some children cry from crossness and some giggle, but none are frightened by this approach.

When your child is almost asleep it's difficult to judge whether to go in again for another kiss. Again it's up to you, but remember that you have made a contract with your child – you'll kiss him in a minute if his head is on the mattress. Maybe it's worth the risk of rousing him just one more time so that he's completely secure about the programme.

The programme requires a lot of energy and time initially, but it can be enjoyable for parents and baby alike, in spite of the sore lips! Be prepared to give up to 300 kisses on the first night over a three-hour period and remember to put your dressing gown on when you get up at night, because you could be busy for some time and feeling cold is a powerful disincentive to seeing it through. Gradually, it will take less time and fewer kisses for your baby to sleep.

As with the controlled crying approach, some children test their parents' resolve – often on night five. If you can weather that storm, the next couple of nights should be the last on the programme. Most children are sleeping easily within a week.

If kisses seem to take too long or your back can't manage all that bending, then a pat on the hand or the head works just as well. Just make the same sort of contact each time.

Sometimes parents live in ways that make this sort of intensive procedure difficult to do. If you are a single parent, start the programme on a Friday, and ask a friend or your mother to have the baby for Saturday and Sunday afternoon so you can sleep. By then your baby should be falling asleep more quickly.

Kate used the kissing game with Jade when, at 18 months, she seemed frightened to go in her cot.

> Jade suddenly stopped wanting to go to bed, it was as if she was scared that if she touched the mattress she would disappear. I didn't know how to go from pacing up and down to putting her down. At the 18-month check-up I told the health visitor all about it and she told me about the kiss-and-retreat programme. The first night they think it's a game so they play along with it until they doze off. The second night they fight it. When she has a tantrum it's really upsetting to watch because she head-butts the wall. She was scooting down to the end of the bed and I was trying to put her back up to the pillow. It was 45 minutes to one hour of constant head-butting and screaming, she was so tired at the end of it she just conked out. On the third night she tried everything she could. But it worked because after a week I stood by the door, and after that outside the door. Then I shut the door and she called to me and I said: "Go to sleep, I'm here." And after that I thought I might as well go downstairs, so I did and she was fine.

Angela and Neil used the same approach with Alex when he was eight months old:

'The problem was that I'd lay there for ages rocking him. He'd sleep for 20 minutes and be awake again. I was up four or five times a night. He basically catnapped. I ended up sleeping with him in the double bed. The health visitor gave me a plan: put him in his cot, give him a kiss, shut the curtains, say "Night-night", and walk away. When he starts creating go back and comfort him. Don't make eye contact. Drop the side of the cot, put my body-weight on him. Say "Everything's OK, mummy's here". The first night was horrendous. It took me an hour each time he woke, straightening the bedding, no eye contact. I sat on the end of the bed with my back to him and then gently worked that bit further out of the room. But it only took about two nights. He went from going to bed at 11pm, and then up at 12, 2am, 4am, and 6am with two catnaps in the morning and three in the afternoon to 40 minutes in the morning, two to two-and-a-half hours in the afternoon, tea, a play, and then upstairs for a long bath, a regular routine in his room for a bottle, and a book. He's usually in bed by about 8pm and sleeps through until 7am or 8am. He's definitely happier during the day and he doesn't look like Count Dracula any more with his red eyes and white face.

If you'd like to try this approach with the support of your health visitor, it's worth showing her a copy of an article by Dr Olwen Wilson who devised the programme. (See the further reading section on page 155 for a complete reference which you can order through your local library.)

Option 4: Gradual Withdrawal

This is the option for you if you don't want your child to cry at all. It's based on the idea that a series of small changes is easier to get used to than one large one. The idea is to distance yourself gradually from your child as he goes to sleep, only moving further away when your child has got used to the previous position.

Take it in tiny stages. If you're lying down with your baby to get him to sleep, sit on the edge of the bed instead, and then when he's happy with that, move to a chair by the bed. Then move the chair little by little across the room. Finally sit outside his door for a few evenings, just so that he can call to you if he needs to. After that you should be able to get on with your evening. Each position may take two or three nights. Don't rush it. Go at the pace your baby can manage. You will need to offer your baby a lot of reassurance that he can manage each new position. If you stay firm it will work.

Some parents find that they begin gradually and are able to speed up the process later. Marion used this technique to get Richard to sleep alone:

When Richard was four I was still lying with him to get him to sleep. I was happy with the arrangement but Richard's sister, Barbara, who was eight, wasn't. She felt it was unfair, because I didn't lie with her. I suppose I might have gone on lying with him but for two or three chance events. Firstly, one night James put Richard to bed and came down after the usual half an hour saying that he had lain on the sofa in the children's room, instead of on Richard's bed because he had a book he wanted to read and Richard hadn't been upset, but had fallen asleep in the same way as usual. So I tried the same approach and it worked.

Then James was offered a job at the other end of the country and had to furnish a flat within a few days, so he needed the sofa from the children's room. Having nothing now to lie on and being a single parent during the week I had to readjust the sleeping arrangements. I told Richard that I needed to spend half an hour with Barbara after he went to bed and that I would just be downstairs if he needed me. It worked amazingly well. I came down after the statutory two songs and a chat, Richard went to sleep and Barbara got some quality time alone with me which she had never had before.

Use the gradual withdrawal approach to move your baby from your bed to his own. But this time it's him rather than you who moves a little further away every two or three nights. On the first night try putting him in his cot with the side down, or on a mattress on the floor next to your bed; after that raise the side on his cot and leave him sleeping next to your bed a little longer. Then gradually begin to move the cot or mattress further across the room and finally into his own room. You can have as many stages on the route to his bedroom as you like.

Variations on a Theme

All these approaches have good points and bad points. Generally, the quickest results mean the most tears. Whichever you choose, stick with it for at least three nights, be prepared for a test night, and be consistent. Some parents have adapted the behavioural approach to fit in with the sort of relationship they have with their children, and feel it works. One mother kept her baby in her bed but patted her back instead of feeding her:

When Hannah was 27 months I decided to stop breastfeeding her as it was starting to annoy me. I couldn't sit down without her being attached to me. We couldn't even look at books together. Firstly, I stopped feeding her in the day. That was the easiest. I just didn't sit down and we went out a lot! After a couple of weeks it was going quite well so I decided to stop her feeding in the night too. When she woke up I lay in her bed next to her (firmly on my front!) and patted her on the back until she went to sleep. After a few days she didn't ask for a feed at bedtime so I decided that was the time to stop altogether.

Dawn, mother of Rebecca, six, Hannah, four, and Lucy 18 months

Another mother, Kim, knew what would work for her third baby, Eden:

We've started a sleep routine now that Pete's got a clear stretch at work. The old routine was that I breastfed Eden until she eventually fell asleep on me. Then she might get up and play for a bit, and then I'd feed her again, she played again – she kept going until she was really tired. Yesterday we went upstairs and looked at her brother and sister in bed and asleep. Then we went into her room and read a story, and she lay down and went to sleep with me stroking her hand. She slept for six hours.

At 2am I went in and stroked her hand for six minutes until she calmed down and went out for a couple of minutes. When I went back in she was standing up and I talked to her about the teddies. I had a resigned calm about me – I didn't force her, I knew I was going to do it. In my heart of hearts I didn't want to be separated from her, but I've had to decide for all our health that I need to do it. I carried on leaving her for two minutes and going in for six. It took 40 minutes. In the end I left her for five minutes and she went off. She woke up at 6am and I brought her into my bed. I felt it was long enough to have gone without a feed.

Just occasionally a baby cries so hard he vomits

We were assured that the controlled crying technique would only take two weeks. But it was terrible. It was barbaric. Both her and our suffering was indescribable. She would scream for hours, bang her head against the cot, pull out her hair, stick her fingers down her throat and make herself sick and, worst of all, cut the inside of her mouth with her nails so that when we went in there would be blood dripping from her mouth.

Fiona, mother of Phoebe

Even more rare and more worrying still is the baby who passes out when he cries. In both cases it's a good idea to visit your GP once again to rule out physical causes for these reactions (or see Chapter 10 on alternative help). If you still want to try a behavioural approach, try a more gradual one, so that your baby doesn't become so upset.

Making it Work
Charts: One for Both of You

Many parents find it helpful to carry on charting their progress, while using a behavioural programme. The sleep diary is a good way to do this. It can be reassuring for you if you're finding the programme difficult, and it can help you to see where the weak points are in your strategy when you feel like giving in. It can also be useful to discuss your chart with the professional or friend who is supporting you.

Your toddler may find star charts exciting. Copy the one below or make your own.

Star chart

Goal: e.g. Jo goes to sleep alone ☺   e.g. Sam stays in his bed ☺

Start date:

	Fri	Sat	Sun	Mon	Tue	Wed	Thur
Week 1	☺	☺	☺	☺			
Week 2							
Week 3							
Week 4							
Week 5							
Week 6							

Either buy some stickers or draw on a star for each night your child achieves the goal you set. Some children like to put up their own sticker, or choose which colour pen you use to draw the star.

Do it as soon as your toddler wakes and make a point of praising him at the same time. If you have had a bad night just ignore the star chart. Don't underline his failure by drawing attention to it and don't give a sticker just to make him feel better – giving a 'free' one diminishes his effort in gaining the others.

You may find that the sticker alone is motivation enough for your child. But some children lose interest after three or four stickers so it may be worth building in a small present or a treat once you are sure that the star chart is beginning to work. However, don't mention the treat before you see which way the wind blows because failing to get a star is one thing, but failing to get a present is another. When you are convinced that your child will make progress with this scheme, offer him a present if he keeps up the good work for just three or four more days. In this way the star chart acts as a motivator and a reward.

Try not to use the star chart to threaten your child at night. If he is finding the programme hard work, it won't make it any easier for him to do it if you say: 'Right then, you've got up again, there's no star for you in the morning.' This will only leave him with a double anxiety – that he must go to sleep alone and yet not get a star. Whatever you do in the morning, you then lose. If you give him a star he may think he can get up each night; if you don't give him one he will believe that he went to sleep on his own for nothing.

It's better to avoid talking about the star chart altogether unless you can do it in a positive way. For example: 'Which sticker are you going to choose tomorrow – a rainbow or a Mickey Mouse?' Or 'Can you remember what you get in the morning when you go to sleep nicely?' Or 'You only have to get one more sticker and then we can go swimming/buy that toy/have your friend to play.'

Climbing Out of Bed

It's easier to help your cot-bound baby to learn to go to sleep alone because he has to stay where he is. When faced with a new bedtime routine many toddlers protest by getting out of bed and coming to find you.

There are three behavioural ways you can help your child learn to stay in his bed.

Game-Plan 1: Back to Bed

If your child gets out of bed, lead him back straight away and without comment. If you are trying a gradual withdrawal approach or the kissing game, then carry on with the same approach as though nothing had happened. If you are trying a cold turkey or controlled crying approach, leave his bedroom once you've put him to bed again and sit outside his door. In this way the back-to-bed routine will be quicker and less frustrating than if you tried to watch television or eat dinner. If you are following the cold turkey plan, continue to sit outside his door until he falls asleep; with the controlled crying plan, return to him only when it is the set time to do so (use the timing charts from page 116). Try to put him back to bed without shouting or forcing him, no matter how tired or frustrated you are. Your child may find these emotional reactions rewarding, and stay awake just to hear you shout some more.

> I recently resolved the bedtime nonsense with Alice (nearly three years old). I told her she was going to learn to go to sleep. I put her in her bed, then sat outside her room. Each time she got up I put her back without a fuss or a row, tucked her in and told her "Goodnight". The first night it was three hours before she stopped coming out – as she got tired, the visits became more frequent! Within ten days she had stopped coming out and only rarely does so now. It was fairly painless. Things improved when we resolved to improve them and gave ourselves a time limit (two weeks), and stuck to it. This is very hard to do when you are exhausted and worn down.

Gillian

Max, who has a rare antibody deficiency which causes him severe pain, used to wake between eight and 15 times a night. But Catherine and Trevor tried the same approach as Gillian:

> The sleep therapist told us that part of Max's sleep problem had been caused by the pain Max experienced and part was the result of the perfectly understandable things we'd done to help him cope with the pain. She was marvellous, she advised us to wait until Max had a spell of being fit and then tackle the part of the sleeping problems that were to do with us. We put him to bed and then sat outside his door. Every time he came out we put him back to bed. We had to keep a record of how many times it happened. Max broke all the records. The first night he got up 217 times in two hours! (Our sleep therapist was amazed – before that the worst case had only been 84 times.) The next night it was much better – only a hundred and something. Within the week he was staying in bed.

Game-Plan 2: Back to Bed and Close the Door (for use with the cold turkey or controlled crying approaches)

Do the same as in game-plan 1 above, but this time tell your child that you are going to close the door and keep it closed for one minute. Tell him that if he is still in bed when you open the door you will leave it open and come and see him when the time is up, if he is out of his bed then you will shut the door for two minutes. Every time your child is still out of bed when you open the door close it again for a minute longer than you did last time. It may be hard for your child to understand all this at once. So you could just say, 'Get into bed, I'll open the door in a minute'.

The only trouble with this approach is the undignified battles you may have with the door handle: you and your toddler on opposite sides of the door pushing and pulling. If you find yourself in this position, give thanks that you have such a tenacious child, but that you are still physically stronger than he is.

Game-Plan 3: Door Fixed Ajar (for use with the cold turkey or controlled crying approaches)

This solution is recommended by Dr Christopher Green in his book *Toddler Taming* (1995). He calls it the rope trick. Many children are frightened when their bedroom door is shut at night, but nevertheless make a habit of coming out. You could try tying the door with some string so that it is just ajar. The gap you leave should be small enough to stop them squeezing out but wide enough to allow sufficient light to enter the room. It is imperative that if you choose this method of controlling your child's wanderings, you make the gap too small for him to force his head through and get it stuck. Make the gap too large and this technique can be dangerous.

Alternatively, a stair gate fixed across the bedroom door can work well unless your child can climb over it. Move away any objects from the doorway that could be climbed.

Ten Point Plan for Success

- Keep a sleep diary for a week before you start.
- Agree your goal. Sleep all night long? Go to sleep on his own? Stay in his own bed all night?
- Agree your method: cold turkey/controlled crying/kisses/gradual withdrawal/other.
- Agree exactly how you will do it: what will you say?/How will you say it?
- Agree who will do it: taking turns every night/one night off—one night on. If you are a lone parent, ask a friend or your mother to help.
- Tell the neighbours what you are doing.
- Explain the programme to your child if appropriate.
- Pick the right time: start the programme when you can afford to be more tired than usual, or can go to bed earlier than usual, when there are no other changes in your baby's life, and no one is ill.
- Keep a record and talk about it to each other or to someone else you trust.
- Try for at least three nights.

And ... enjoy your sleep, and a happy child in the morning, eventually!

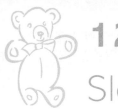

12

Sleeping at the Wrong Time

The behaviour management approach can also be used to solve sleeping problems caused when your baby sleeps at the wrong time of day.

Late Bedtimes and Late Risers

Late bedtimes and late wakings are common among children and adolescents. They can also occur as part of other sleep problems in younger children. It is tempting to allow a child who has a late bedtime to sleep late in the morning, so that you can have some time to yourself. But if you would like your evening without your child, then you will have to adjust the time he gets up. Very few children sleep for 14 hours at a stretch.

The easiest way to do this is to wake your child a little earlier every morning so that his night is cut short and he is ready for bed at an increasingly early time. Begin by allowing him two more days of late bedtimes but without any attempt to bring them earlier. Make a record of when he wakes. The morning after the third night, wake him 15–30 minutes earlier than he woke the previous mornings. Do this for the next three days as well, bringing the waking time earlier by 15–30 minutes each day without changing the bedtime.

Once your child is having 45 or 60 minutes less sleep than usual each night, start to make bedtime 15–30 minutes earlier each night. At the same time continue to wake your child progressively earlier until he is getting up at a convenient time. Once you reach the preferred waking time, stick to it every day, even at weekends, for the next few months until the pattern is firmly established. The same goes for bedtime.

During this programme your child will be mildly sleep deprived. Try not to let him nap during the day any more than normal or he won't be ready for bed by the right time.

Daytime Naps

Some settling problems arise when a baby has a late afternoon nap, and is just not sleepy. If your baby still needs his sleep, move the nap progressively earlier in the day, say by ten minutes each day. You could also try to shorten his nap by ten minutes each week. If he is more than one year old he may be fine on just one nap a day. Try dropping the afternoon nap and re-scheduling the morning nap to straddle lunchtime by moving it on by ten minutes every two or three days.

Sometimes difficulties arise when a child gives up his daytime nap, usually between two and three years old. For a few months the lack of a nap can mean that your child becomes overtired by the evening and is therefore overactive and stressed. Being overtired can also cause more waking at night. If so, don't wait until he is sleepy before beginning your bedtime routine, he may be too tired to cope with it and may resist sleep when he's put into his cot. Try starting half an hour earlier than you usually do.

Another solution is to let your child keep his daytime sleep but encourage him to sleep earlier than before and wake him after he has had half the usual time. You may find that he doesn't want to sleep at the time that would suit you; if so, encourage him to rest, lying down on his bed, perhaps looking at books.

Early Risers

This is one of the most intractable sleep problems.

> For early wakening, nothing works. We tried blackouts, later bedtimes and no naps in the day, but nothing works.
> **Diana**

Many children just seem to rise with the sun no matter what you do or how late they go to bed. But there are various approaches that may help.

Your child could be waking because he knows that something good happens when he does. Such a thirst for life might actually be engaging if 5am didn't come quite so early in the morning. Perhaps you always slot a video in when you come down and you feel too tired to play. Even a feed or a cuddle as soon as he wakes could be rewarding.

If your baby is still in a cot, try delaying any reward until a little later each morning, gradually increasing the time that he must wait, say, five minutes longer the first morning and then ten minutes after three days. However, if your baby wakes you by crying every morning, you may have to take a different tack first. Crying gets the day off to a bad start. So, go in before he cries, smile and show him that you're happy he's awake. Once you've done this for a week he should be sure that you'll come before he's desperate so you can begin to delay going to him for those few minutes.

Continue to increase the delay until you reach half an hour. You may find that after about ten days he is sleeping longer in the morning, and then you can start the delaying process again. But don't try it too many times – some children are just happy and awake in the morning. If you are putting your one-year-old to sleep at 6pm you shouldn't be surprised if he is awake by 6am the following morning.

Once your child can now climb out of his cot you'll need to go to him quickly in the morning or move him into a bed. Alternatively, something external could be waking him. Central heating timers, early morning commuters, milk deliveries or sunshine could all have an effect. You could try switching the heating on later, moving your child to another room or installing secondary glazing, buying your milk at the supermarket or black-out blinds.

 Cara had a lot of sleep problems, and she's still not a brilliant sleeper. I think some people just aren't. She used to cry in the night, and wake early. We didn't do anything very clever about the early waking. We tried black-out blinds, but they didn't work. It was her body clock that was waking her up, not the light outside. She used to be up at about 5am or 5.30am, but I refused to get up until 6.30am. She'd just lie in her cot, and presumably she'd had enough sleep by then, so she was happy enough. We refused to have her in our bed, because we knew that we wouldn't sleep, and anyway we thought that at some point she has to sort this out for herself. We didn't try putting her to bed later – she always went at about 7pm. But we expected her to sleep 12 hours, but she never did. We didn't worry about it, because she wasn't our first, so we knew we weren't doing anything wrong. Now, at seven years old, she still gets up early, but entertains herself.

Hilary and Mike

You can also use the behavioural approach at the end of the day to address this problem. Try putting your child to bed progressively later each night by about 15 minutes so that after a few days he is waking later. But do not let him nap more than usual during the day.

Some children have what sleep counsellor Mary Kasper calls a 'detached nap' – an early morning sleep, only two or three hours after an early waking. These sleeps may be handy for parents, because while the baby naps they can get the older children off to playgroup or school or organize themselves for the day. But if the early morning waking is a problem, the solution lies in joining that early morning nap back to the night-time sleep.

You can do this by gradually delaying the nap by a few minutes each day so that it stops being a top-up for the night and becomes 'fully detached'. Your child should spontaneously start to sleep longer in the mornings. Watch out for him being ready for bed earlier than usual and ensure that you stick to a bedtime that is convenient.

Many early risers grow out of the condition when they begin playgroup or school, and if they don't then by this age they are able to entertain themselves more easily for a short time without waking you. A drink and a biscuit placed with a few interesting toys next to your toddler's bed, ready for the morning, may give you a couple more minutes' grace.

If none of this works, you may have to resign yourself to an early start to your day. Go to bed earlier yourself and make the most of the mornings. There's something virtuous about rising before anyone else, which can make you feel pleasantly superior for hours at a time.

Toddlers and older children respond quite well to being told that they can get up/come into parent's bed when they hear the alarm clock. Start by setting the alarm for the approximate time that your child wakes then gradually set it 5–10 minutes later each day until an acceptable time is reached. This can be combined with a star chart (page 126).

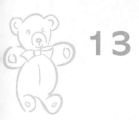

13

Beyond Babies

Most of this book is about babies and children under two years. But sleep problems don't disappear when your baby becomes a toddler. Older children can have some of the same problems and may develop a whole new collection to keep you amused as they develop.

Nightmares and Night Terrors

Most children have nightmares at one time or another, but far fewer have night terrors. Nightmares and night terrors are different things and require dramatically different handling.

Nightmares

Nightmares are four times more common than night terrors. They tend to affect children of three to four years old and eight to ten years old, particularly boys, although some children as young as two have them occasionally. Children who sleep in the same bed or the same room as their parents have fewer nightmares.

Nightmares are common when your child is developing rapidly, gaining a new sense of awareness about the world. At age three to four your child is asking 'why?' a lot, and at age eight to ten he is beginning to understand general principles. Children also have more nightmares when they are anxious. They are not necessarily a sign of emotional disturbance – it's just as likely that a scary story or a film before bed is to blame.

Nightmares usually happen when your child is dreaming, in the lightest sleep state, in the final third of the night. Your child will call out and will be obviously upset. He will be awake and can remember the dream, although little children may find it hard to describe.

Your child may sleep more easily if you give him explanations that he can understand to his many questions during the day. If nightmares occur often, make time for an especially peaceful bedtime routine, with a lot of reassurance and cuddling, a night light or a special toy.

Night Terrors

Night terrors are rare. They affect only about 5% of children, usually boys aged between four and seven, and they often run in families. Night terrors come and go with regular episodes followed by long peaceful intervals. There are no long- or short-term effects of night terrors.

They usually occur when your child is coming out of the deepest part of sleep, in the first three hours of sleep. The part of the brain that affects the expression of emotion wakes, but the part that is related to memory and awareness remains deeply asleep. This means that your child may look as though he is having a truly horrific experience but he won't remember a thing in the morning, or even immediately after the night terror if he is brought to full awakening.

Night terrors begin with a piercing scream. Your child will be sitting in bed, staring ahead, possibly sweating or mumbling incoherently. He will not appear to be aware of his surroundings or of you. He will not be awake and will resist being woken.

> Harry would wake up an hour after he had gone to sleep and sit bolt upright. He didn't want to be comforted. It would almost be as if he was blind – as if he couldn't see you – it seemed as if he was in the middle of a nightmare. The night terrors used to happen if he missed his afternoon sleep – because he was overtired, and couldn't shift from one sort of sleep to another.

Ann

Stay, if you like, to put your mind at rest, but let him fall asleep without waking fully. He may push you away if you try to cuddle him – he does not know it is you. Don't question him either then or in the morning – he won't know the answers, but your questioning may worry him. Alternatively, wake your child 15 minutes before the terror usually occurs, at the first sign of increased movement. Within three or four nights you may be able to break the pattern.

> Jessica's sleep terrors were made worse because I was trying to get her to stop crying by holding her and she was fighting me off. Once I learnt to leave her until she came to me, the terrors stopped.

Yvonne

Drugs, such as diazepam, which decrease the amount of time spent in stage 3 and 4 sleep, can be prescribed if the terrors occur nightly and have been present for a long time, but most children grow out of them and drugs are rarely needed.

Sleepwalking

Sleepwalking usually occurs when your child is in the deepest stage of sleep, within the first three hours of falling asleep. Part of your child's brain becomes aroused and part remains deeply asleep. He is able to move but not to be aware of or to remember what he does.

Sleepwalking occurs regularly in 1–15% of children and tends to affect children aged four to eight, particularly boys. If you walked in your sleep as a child, your child is six times more likely than other children to do the same. Some children (about 10%) who sleepwalk also have night terrors. It may be that the same mechanism accounts for both disturbances.

Your sleepwalking child may appear to be looking for something, but he won't be able to tell you what. Sleepwalkers may on occasion eat or dress themselves. It is common for children to be partially aware that they need to wee, but to mistake other objects for the toilet.

Lindsay remembers sleepwalking as a child:

> I know that on one occasion I was walking round the house, and my mother was following me, just watching. I know I got onto a stool and peed on it and my mother was horrified.

Some children sleepwalk nightly and others only when triggered. Triggers may be a full bladder, noise, stress, anxiety, fever or sleep deprivation. Pat's father died suddenly when she was 16:

> I can remember waking up on a swing in the local park where my dad and I used to go a lot when I was little. It was really frightening to find myself out there in my nightie.

Sleepwalking usually only occurs once in a night and for only 15 minutes at a time, ending spontaneously with the child returning to bed and to sleep. Your sleepwalking child will be difficult to wake and in fact it is best not to wake him. Some parents find that they can suggest to their child that he returns to bed and others can lead their child there but if your child doesn't go, don't force him.

It is possible for your child to injure himself while he is sleepwalking. If he sleepwalks regularly, don't let him sleep in the top bunk or have mirrors in his room, clear the floor and the stairs of toys and, if he is young, put up a stair gate. Ensure that all windows are locked at night and that the front door is secured with a high lock.

Most young sleepwalkers gradually grow out of it. For older children and teenagers, sleepwalking and night terrors may indicate unresolved emotional stresses. If your child is having frequent episodes you may like to consult your doctor for medication or counselling. Drug treatment (diazepam) is available for long, frequent episodes but is not usually needed, and should be seen only as a temporary measure.

Bed Wetting (Enuresis)

Bed wetting can make you feel very frustrated and angry, but it is important that you don't direct this at your child. If your child feels embarrassed or ashamed of his bed wetting, these feelings may become a longer lasting and more damaging experience than the bed wetting in itself will ever be.

Bed wetting at night may become a problem for you when your child continues to wet at night after all his contemporaries have become dry. If it continues it may become a problem for him because you may not feel able to allow him to stay away over night with friends.

> Naomi was out of nappies in the day early on. And at three-and-a-half was out of nappies at night. But right up until Christmas last year when she was seven, she had wet beds four or five times a week. She was quite unconcerned about it and even happy to tell her peers that she wet. From our point of view it wasn't a problem. When she was little we used to lift her for a wee, but we stopped doing that as she got bigger. The school nurse asked me if it was still a problem for us and I said, "Well, it's not a problem because we have a washing machine." Since Christmas she's only wet four times, so it obviously wasn't a mechanical problem.

Jane

Sometimes your child will start bed wetting again after being dry. Sometimes this happens when he feels under stress. A house move, the birth of a new baby, the death of a relative or a new school can all be stressful. If you can help him to talk about his worries, the bed wetting may fade away.

Most children are dry by four-and-a-half years old, but some, especially children with a mental or physical disability, take longer, and the most seriously disabled never learn. Your GP will treat it as a problem only when your child is five years old or more.

Ask your GP to check your child of over five years for physical problems which may cause his bed wetting (physical causes are often the culprit when your child has been dry for a few months and then begins to wet again). Physical causes may include urinary infections, diabetes, allergies or sleep apnoea (breathing pauses).

Once you have ruled out physical problems, you could try a behavioural approach. Use a star chart to reward your child for every dry night (see page 126 for details of how to use one). Continue with the star chart until your child has two months of dry nights with only the occasional accident. You can use the star chart alone or in combination with a programme in which you train your child to wait for longer before he urinates.

Training Programme

In the early evening encourage your child to drink a lot. When he is ready to urinate ask him to wait for five minutes, and then let him go. If he fails to wait, reassure him and ask him to try the same thing again the next time he is ready. If he does manage to wait, praise him for his control. Once he has successfully waited five minutes on three different occasions, ask him to wait ten minutes. Each time he succeeds in waiting the time you have asked three times, increase the time he must wait by five minutes until you have reached half an hour. Encourage your child to go to the toilet before he goes to bed for the night. The next night do the same again, but if he was easily able to wait five minutes the previous night, ask him to wait ten minutes this time. Continue this drinking and waiting programme for three weeks.

The programme will help your child to increase his bladder control and learn the correct signals for urination.

While you are carrying out the programme, encourage your child to practise stopping and starting the urine flow while on the toilet at least once a day.

After three weeks stop plying your child with drink but ask him to wait for half an hour before he urinates. In the last five minutes of the allotted time ask him to lay down in his darkened bedroom as though he were going to sleep. Tell him to count to 20 before he gets up and goes to the bathroom. Let him sit on the toilet, but ask him not to urinate. Ask him to do this ten times before he finally urinates. At each point in the training programme praise your child if he succeeds, or reassure your child if he fails to wait the desired time, but ask him to try again. Continue with this for three weeks.

If this doesn't work, see your GP again and ask him for a 'bell and pad' apparatus. This is an electrical device which rings when your child begins to wet and wakes him. It is completely safe but may take between three and six months to work.

> We saw someone about it before Isaac was seven because I was so desperate, but maybe we shouldn't have, because you lose the momentum. Isaac's nine now and we're down to a wet once a week from six times in a week, using a pad and bell apparatus from the school nurse. But we've had dry periods before and it's all gone to pieces when we remove the pad and bell. First of all we want to get to no wets and then we want to be able to remove the pad and bell. It's not something that will be solved overnight. He doesn't seem bothered about it usually, but occasionally he says "Mummy, when am I going to be dry?" and every night in his prayers he asks God to help him to be dry. When we first started a star chart I had to stop him running out into the street to tell everyone – I didn't want him inadvertently getting himself teased. It's extremely frustrating when you have night after night after night of wet beds. You feel helpless as a parent because you can't do that bit for your child. You can provide all the stimulants and aids, but you can't do that bit.

Charlotte, mother of four

If all else fails, your doctor may prescribe your child a drug called desmopressin to help control the problem.

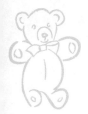

14

Afterthought

Sometimes, no matter what you do, your child doesn't want to sleep when you want him to. It happens. But if you have tried everything, maybe now is a good time to just accept it. Acceptance won't make the problem disappear but it may make it easier to bear. One parent's problem is another's good night. Here's what other parents have found.

 The biggest problem comes when you try to fight them – you can't fight the fundamental pattern.

Cathy, mother of two

 If I ever have a dilemma about how to deal with a parenting problem I ask myself what I would do if I hadn't read any books or heard any one else's opinions. I think there is a huge learning curve in parenting but with each extra child you have, the more your experience can help you do better. I think each family has to work it out for themselves.

Dawn, mother of three

> We tried leaving him to cry, it never worked, giving him drugs, that didn't work, taking turns, putting him in our bed, watching videos, driving round in the car, laying with him while he went to sleep and musical beds but only sleeping with him worked – he just wanted company. Children grow out of it eventually. Accept them for what they are – only little. We cannot control everything in our lives but we can adapt to sleep disturbances.

Diana, mother of three

> I'd say to other parents that it will happen, eventually. Jennifer was six when she finally slept a night in her own bed for the first time. If you can't stomach behaviour management methods, just wait patiently, keep your sense of humour and keep trying. At seven years Jennifer is our most confident/sociable/outward going/peer group loving child. After not being separated from us without a HUGE FUSS for six long years she finally severed the cord and FLEW. I like to think (and this makes it all worth while) that if we'd "sleep cliniced"/drugged or otherwise forced her to separate from us before she was ready, it would have made a detrimental difference to her development.

Ann, mother of four

> When you have a baby you just accept that they wake in the night and deal with it, knowing it doesn't last forever.

Dawn, mother of six

Tips for Getting Through the Night ...

- Accept it
- Know it doesn't last
- Concentrate on the good bits
- Turn the clock to the wall – does it really matter what time it is?
- Take turns each hour/each night
- Do whatever makes it easier

... and the Day

- Slow down
- Sleep whenever you can

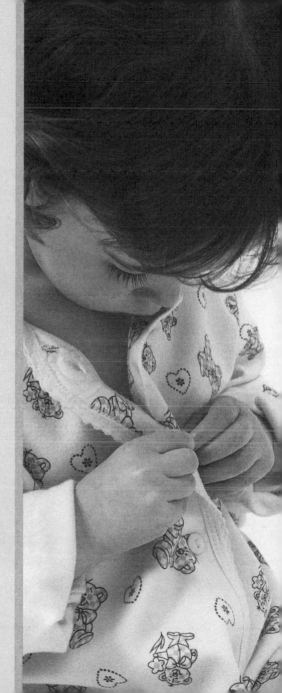

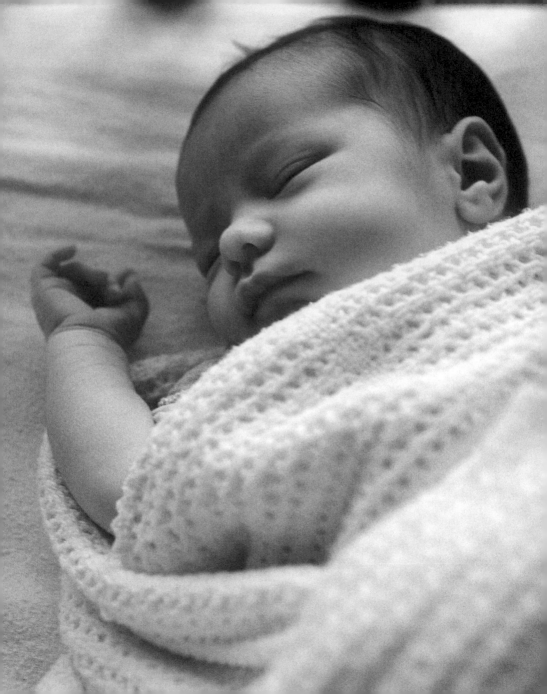

Resources

ORGANIZATIONS

SERENE/CRY-sis
Support for families with
excessively crying, sleepless and
demanding children.

BM CRY-sis
London WC1N 3XX
CRY-sis helpline 0207 404 5011
Operates from 8am to 11pm,
seven days a week.

ParentlinePlus
Support and information for all
families (incorporating Parent
Network courses on parenting
skills).

ParentlinePlus
520 Highgate Studios
53–79 Highgate Road
Kentish Town
London NW5 1TL
Helpline 0207 284 5000
www.parentlineplus.org.uk

Meet-A-Mum Association
(MAMA)
MAMA organizes local groups
offering friendship and support to
mothers who feel isolated or have
postnatal depression

Helpline 0208 768 0123
Operates from 7pm to 10pm
weekdays (10am to 1pm on
Mondays and Wednesdays).

The Foundation for the Study of Infant Deaths (FSID)
Information about avoiding cot death.

FSID
Artillery House
11–19 Artillery Row
London SW1P 1RT
Tel: 0207 222 8001
Fax: 0207 222 8002

BRIEF PSYCHOANALYTIC THERAPY

(see page 103 for a description)

Contact one of the organizations below in the first instance to find out more and then, if it sounds like what you need, ask your GP to refer you.

Child Psychotherapy Trust
The CPT have a series of leaflets on emotional development and baby behaviour, and relationships to parents, such as 'Your New Baby' and 'Crying and Sleeping'. These cost £1 each and are available from the CPT at:

Child Psychotherapy Trust
Star House
104–108 Grafton Road
London NW5 4BD
Tel: 0207 284 1355
E-mail: cpt@globalnet.co.uk
Please enclose an A4 SAE to cover postage.

Association of Child Psychotherapists
Contact the ACP for the name of a registered child psychotherapist near you. Child psychotherapists are available privately and through the NHS.

Association of Child Psychotherapists
120 West Heath Road
London NW3 7TU
Tel: 0208 458 1609

COMPLEMENTARY PRACTITIONERS

Acupuncture

For a list of registered acupuncturists who have trained to work with children, contact:

June Tranmer MBAcC
Practitioner of Paediatric Acupuncture
The Healing Clinic
33 Fulford Cross
York YO10 4PB
Tel: 01904 679868

Cranial Osteopathy

Osteopathic Centre for Children
109 Harley Street
London W1G 6AN
Tel: 0207 486 6160
Website: www.cranial.org.uk

Homoeopathy

For a full list of doctors trained in homoeopathy, an information pack and NHS availability, send an SAE to:

British Homoeopathic Association
15 Clerkenwell Close
London EC1R 5AA
Tel: 0207 566 7800

Baby Massage

For details of baby massage classes and qualified baby masseurs near you, contact:

International Association of Infant Massage (UK Office)
56 Sparsholt Road,
Barking Essex IG11 7YQ
Tel: 07816 289788 (10.30am to 2.30pm)
E-mail: mail@iaim.org.uk

Intrinsic Development

This new approach is the work of Pam Stretch, a physiotherapist and reflex therapist who has been developing it in India and here for the last 10 years. For more information, write to:

Pam Stretch
23 Yew Tree Road
Ormskirk
Lancashire L39 1NS

Attention Deficit Hyperactivity
Disorder (ADHD)
Hyperactive Children's Support
Group
71 Whyke Lane
Chichester
PO19 2LD
Tel: 01234 551313

For information not covered here,
ring the National Childbirth Trust
Enquiry Line on 0870 444 8707
and they should be able to
recommend an organization that
can help you.

SUPPLIERS

Slings

There are many different designs
of sling for carrying your baby on
your front, hip or back, suitable
for babies from birth onwards. If
you intend to use the sling from
birth, check that it will provide
sufficient support for your baby's
head. Slings are available from
any baby equipment shop or by
mail order from the small
advertizements in any baby
magazine.

NCT Maternity Sales

Find a good selection of baby
equipment and gifts to buy from
the National Childbirth Trust by
phone on 0141 636 0600 or online
at www.nctms.co.uk

John Lewis stores stock the
following:

Brio Wonderland Bed-Side-Cot

A cot with a removable side and
adjustable base that can be fixed
to abut your own bed. The Bed-
Side-Cot provides your baby with
his own sleep space within easy
reach for night-time feeds.

The Swinging Cradle

A cradle that you rock by hand.
Suitable for babies from birth to
four months, depending on the
weight of your baby.

The Baby Swing

A swing for babies with a seat
similar to a car-seat in which your
baby can be rocked for 15 minutes
at a time. Suitable for babies
aged four to nine months.

Website: www.johnlewis.com

Further Reading

Books

Daws, D. (1993) *Through the Night*, Free Association Books, London.

Douglas, J. and Richman, N. (1984) *My Child Won't Sleep*, Penguin, London.

Ferber, R. (1985) *Solve Your Child's Sleep Problems: The Complete Practical Guide for Parents*, Dorling Kindersley, London.

Green, C. (1995) *Toddler Taming: A Parent's Guide to the First Four Years*, Ebury Press, London.

Haslam, D. (1992) *Sleepless Children: A Handbook for Parents*, Piatkus, London.

Henderson, A. (1997) *The Good Sleep Guide*, ABC Health Guides, Corsham.

Hollyer, B. and Smith, L. (1996) *Sleep. The Secret of Problem-free Nights*, Ward Lock, London.

Jackson, D. (1989) *Three in a Bed: Why You Should Sleep With Your Baby*, Bloomsbury, London.

Liedloff, J. (1989) *The Continuum Concept*, Arkana, London.

Quine, L. (1997) *Solving Children's Sleep Problems*, Beckett Karlson, Cambridge.

St James-Roberts, I., Harris, G. and Messer, D. (eds) (1993) *Infant Crying, Feeding and Sleeping*, Harvester Wheatsheaf, Hemel Hempstead.

Scott, J. (1990) *Natural Medicine for Children*, Unwin Hyman, London.

Schneider, V. (1989) *Infant Massage: A Handbook for Loving Parents*, Bantam, USA (available from Yolande Bosman Therapies and Training, tel: 0115 982 0389).

Sears, W. and M. (1995) *Little Angels: Everything You Need to Know to have a Better-behaved Child – From Birth to Ten Years*, Hodder & Stoughton, London.

Thevenin, T. (1987) *The Family Bed: An Age-old Concept in Child-Rearing*, Avery.

Articles

Anders, T. (1978) as cited in Messer, D. and Richards, M. (1993) 'The development of sleeping difficulties', in I. St James-Roberts, G. Harris and D. Messer (eds) *Infant Crying, Feeding and Sleeping*, Harvester Wheatsheaf, Hemel Hempstead, p. 151.

Anders, T.F., Keener, M.A. and Kraemer, H. (1985) as cited in Z. Zaiwalla and A. Stein (1993) 'The physiology of sleep in infants', in I. St James-Roberts, G. Harris and D. Messer (eds) *Infant Crying, Feeding and Sleeping*, Harvester Wheatsheaf, Hemel Hempstead, p. 142.

Beltramini, A.U. and Hertzig, M.E. (1983) as cited in D. Messer and M. Richards (1993) 'The development of sleeping difficulties' in I. St James-Roberts, G. Harris and D. Messer (eds) *Infant Crying, Feeding and Sleeping*, Harvester Wheatsheaf, Hemel Hempstead, p. 155.

Bernal, J. (1972) 'Crying during the first ten days of life, and maternal responses', *Developmental Medicine and Child Neurology*, 14: 362–72.

Billingham, R.E. and Zentall, S. (1996) 'Co-sleeping: gender differences in college students' retrospective reports of sleeping with parents during childhood', *Psychological Reports*, 79, 3 part 2: 1423–6.

Carskadon, M.A. and Dement, W.C. (1989) as cited in Z. Zaiwalla and A. Stein (1993) 'The physiology of sleep in infants' in I. St James-

Roberts, G. Harris and D. Messer (eds) *Infant Crying, Feeding and Sleeping*, Harvester Wheatsheaf, Hemel Hempstead, p. 137.

Durant, V.M. and Mindell, J.A. (1990) 'Behavioural treatment of multiple childhood sleep disorders', *Behaviour Modification*, 14: 37–9.

Lodemore, M., Peterson, S.A. and Wailoo, M.P. (1991) as cited in Z. Zaiwalla and A. Stein (1993) 'The physiology of sleep in infants' in I. St James-Roberts, G. Harris and D. Messer (eds) *Infant Crying, Feeding and Sleeping*, Harvester Wheatsheaf, Hemel Hempstead, p. 142.

McKenna, J., Mosko, S., Richard, C. *et al.* (1994) 'Experimental studies of infant–parent co-sleeping: mutual physiological and behavioural influences and their relevance to SIDS (sudden infant death syndrome)', *Early Human Development*, 38: 187–210.

Messer, D. and Richards, M. (1993) 'The development of sleeping difficulties' in I. St James-Roberts, G. Harris and D. Messer (eds) *Infant Crying, Feeding and Sleeping*, Harvester Wheatsheaf, Hemel Hempstead, p. 151.

Moore, T. and Ucko, L.E. (1957) 'Night waking in early infancy: part 1', *Archives of Disease in Childhood*, 32: 333–43.

Mosko, S., Richards, C., McKenna, J., Drummond, S. and Mukai, D. (1997) 'Maternal proximity and infant CO_2 environment during bedsharing and possible implications for SIDS research', *American Journal of Physical Anthropology*, 103 (3): 315–28.

Rotenberg,V.S. (1992) 'Sleep and memory 1: The influence of different sleep stages on memory' (review), *Neuroscience and Bio-behavioural Reviews*, 16 (4): 497–502.

Scott, G. and Richards, M. (1989) 'Night waking in infants: effects of providing advice and support for parents', *Journal of Child Psychology and Psychiatry*, 31: 551–69.

Wilson, O.H.M. (1996) 'Peace at last: a model of sleep management for parents', *Health Visitor*, 69 (12): 491–2.

Wittig, R.M. and Keenum, A.J. (1997) 'Sleep log data, age seven to 31 months', paper presented at 11th Annual APSS Meeting, 10–15 June, San Francisco, California.

Wolson, A., Lacks, P. and Futterman, A. (1992) 'Effects of parent training on infant sleeping patterns, parents' stress, and perceived parental competence', *Journal of Consulting and Clinical Psychology*, 60 (1): 41–8.

Wright, P., Macleod, H.A. and Cooper, M.J. (1983) 'Waking at night: the effect of early feeding experience', *Child: Care, Health and Development*, 9: 309–19.

The Internet

There's a phenomenal amount of research on sleep accessible through the Internet, but as yet little practical help. I found well over a thousand references when I asked for anything to do with infants and children. If you want to have a browse, the best place to start is:

http://bisleep.medsch.ucla.edu

About the National Childbirth Trust

Run by parents, for parents, the National Childbirth Trust is a self-help charity organization with 400 branches across the UK. There's bound to be a local branch near you, running:

- childbirth classes
- breastfeeding counselling
- new baby groups
- open house get-togethers
- support for dads
- working-parents' groups
- sales of nearly-new baby clothes and equipment

– as well as loads of events where you can meet and make friends with other people going through the same changes.

- To find the contact details of your local branch, ring the NCT Enquiries Line: 0870 444 8707.
- To get support with feeding your baby, ring the NCT Breastfeeding Line: 0870 444 8708. Any day, 8am to 10pm.
- To find answers to pregnancy queries, ring the Enquiries Line or log on to: www.nctpregnancyandbabycare.com

- To buy excellent baby goods, maternity bras, toys and gifts, call 0141 636 0600 or look at: www.nctms.co.uk
- To join the NCT, just call 0870 990 8040 with a credit card.

You don't have to become a member to enjoy the services and support of the National Childbirth Trust. It's open to everyone. We do encourage people to join the charity because it helps fund our work – supporting all parents.

When you become an NCT member and join your local group, you'll get a regular neighbourhood newsletter (a guide to your area aimed at new parents) and you'll also receive NCT's *New Generation* – our mailed-out members' magazine that takes an in-depth look at all issues of interest to new parents.

'The NCT support network is second to none. It's very reassuring and comforting.'

The National Childbirth Trust wants all parents to have an experience of pregnancy, birth and early parenthood that enriches their lives and gives them confidence in being a parent.

National Childbirth Trust
Alexandra House
Oldham Terrace
London W3 6NH
Tel: 0870 770 3236
Fax: 0870 770 3237

Index

massaging the baby 84–5, 151
Meet-A-Mum Association
   (MAMA) 97, 149
mental stimulation 67
mobiles 80
mothers
   feelings of 20–1, 72–5, 89–92
   needs of 17–8
   obtaining REM sleep 9, 11
   and a sense of certainty 13–14
   talking and listening to the
      baby 14–15, 21–4
   see also parents
movement 87–8
music, and crying babies 31, 73

naps
   daytime 26, 27, 121, 133
   and early risers 135–6
   giving up 133
National Childbirth Trust (NCT)
   97, 157
needs
   identifying needs of crying
      babies 77–9
   of parents and babies 17–18,
      23
new-born babies
   and bed-sharing 36–7, 38
   and body temperature 36
   feeding 49–50
   in Japan 42
   and REM sleep 8
   waking at night 5, 60
night lights 83
night terrors 137, 138–9
   and sleepwalking 140
night-time
   amount of sleep needed, and
      age of baby 3
   feeding 48, 53–5
      and help from partners 50,
      57–8
   settling in the evening,
      behaviour management
      plans 114–23

see also bedtime routines;
   waking at night
night-time feeding, stopping
   53–5
nightmares 137, 138
noise 82, 86
NREM sleep 7, 8–9

older children 137–44
   bed wetting (enuresis) 141–4
   night terrors 137, 138–9, 140
   nightmares 137–8, 139
   sleepwalking 140–1
organizations 149–50

pain
   babies crying in 78–9
   babies sucking to relieve
      56–7
   sleep problems as a result of
      104, 128–9
Parent Network 149
parent and toddler groups 97
parents
   acceptance by 145–7
   of children with sleep
      problems 61, 68
   feelings towards the baby
      19–20, 72–5, 89–92
   positive 78
   support groups 103
partners
   and bed-sharing 47
   and bedtime routines 29
   help from 10
   and night feeding 50, 57–8
   relationships with 58, 94–5
   sharing the load with 93–7
   sleeping alone 41, 95–6
   talking to 92–3
Phenergan 100, 101
physical problems, and bed
   wetting 141–2
positive parents 78
postnatal depression 15, 59,
   90

practical problems 16
practical tips 80–8
   company 85–6
   for getting through the night
      147
   heat 81–2
   light 83
   music and movement 86
   noise 82, 86
   for sharing the load 94
   touch 84–5
   toys 80–1
   wrapping snugly 83–4
premature babies 62
   and body temperature 36
   breathing pauses 36
   and REM sleep 8
   waking at night 60–1, 79
promethazine 100
psychoanalytic therapy 103,
   150
pulsatilla 88

'reassurance principle' 96
reflex therapy 67
relaxing, and crying babies
   75–6
REM sleep 7, 8, 9
   deprivation 10
rocking 88
routines
   establishing a routine 13, 59,
      114
   and night-time feeding 54–5
   organizing the day 26–8
   support with establishing a
      new routine 96, 97
   see also bedtime routines

sad babies 78
safe sleeping 33–4
   bed-sharing 40–1
   with door fixed ajar 130
   and sleepwalking 141
self-fulfilling prophecies 68
self-help groups 103

Other titles in the series:

Toddler Tantrums

Penney Hames

Penney Hames explains why children's emotions run strong at this age and shares tried-and-tested methods to help you deal with toddler tantrums.

185 x 150 mm
£6.99
0-00-713609-9

Breastfeeding for Beginners

Caroline Deacon

This guide will provide you with all the help you need to begin breastfeeding and continue successfully.

185 x 150 mm
£6.99
0-00-713608-0

First Foods and Weaning

Ravinder Lilly

Ravinder Lilly answers all your questions about weaning your baby and how to provide a good variety of the right foods using simple recipes.

185 x 150 mm
£6.99
0-00-713607-2

Successful Potty Training

Heather Welford

Helps you spot when your child is ready to move out of nappies and decide on the right method for you both. Includes tips for when you are out and about.

185 x 150 mm
£6.99
0-00-713606-4